ESOPHAGEAL RECONSTRUCTION

Authored by
Marta Strutyńska-Karpińska and
Krzysztof Grabowski

Esophageal Reconstruction
Authored by: **Marta Strutyńska-Karpińska and Krzysztof Grabowski**

Published by InTech

Janeza Trdine 9, 51000 Rijeka, Croatia

Publishing Process Manager Jelena Marušić

Technical Editor InTech DTP Team

Cover Designer InTech Design Team

Additional hard copies can be obtained from orders@intechopen.com

Esophageal Reconstruction
Authored by: Marta Strutyńska-Karpińska and Krzysztof Grabowski
p. cm.
ISBN 978-953-51-0667-8

For EU product safety concerns:
IN TECH d.o.o., Prolaz Marije Krucifikse Kozulić 3, 51000 Rijeka, Croatia,
info@intechopen.com or visit our website at intechopen.com.

Meet the authors

Professor Marta Strutyńska-Karpińska and Professor Krzysztof Grabowski graduated from Medical University in Wrocław. They have worked at the Department and Clinic of Gastrointestinal and General Surgery of Medical University in Wrocław, a unique scientific and clinical center in Poland, which over 30 years, encompasses all aspects of esophageal diseases treatment. Surgery of gastrointestinal tract is of great interest of authors and esophageal surgery occupies the major place. Knowledge, experience and high qualifications in clinical practice they achieved under the guidance of Professor Zdzisław Jezioro and Professor Mieczysław Bernat, their predecessors and teachers. The scientific output of the authors consists of over 400 studies in the field of surgery, among them are 2 books devoted to esophageal surgery.

Contents

Esophageal Reconstruction

Marta Strutyńska-Karpińska
Krzysztof Grabowski

University of Medicine, Department and Clinic
of Gastrointestinal and General Surgery, Skłodowskiej-Curie str. 66,
Wrocław, Poland

Foreword

A significant development of esophageal reconstructive surgery can be observed over the years since 1907, when Cesar Roux first succeeded in performing the esophageal reconstruction with a segment of the jejunum. Professional literature presents both, various modifications of the surgical methods as well as original reconstructive procedures, which broaden significantly the range of surgical modalities and solutions in the surgical management of this condition.

However all the achievements have not led to the development of one, universal and generally accepted surgical method. The main reason of the situation lies in difficulty to standardize reconstructive surgeries. Progress in this respect achieved over time consists mainly in attempts to approximate optimally the function of the reconstructed esophagus to the function of a natural organ, and to minimize the number of both, early and late postsurgical complications.

Success of every reconstructive surgery with the use of pedicled intestinal segment is conditioned by efficient blood supply and adequate length of the pedicle that would enable free from tension anastomosis of the graft with cervical esophagus or the pharynx. Selection of an adequate segment of the intestine for esophageal grafting is in every case closely associated with the anatomical structure of the intestinal vasculature, what means that only the presence of well developed and efficient main blood vessels and their branching arcades may authorize the surgeon to start mobilizing this or another intestinal segment as an esophageal graft. Abandonment of this basic principle leads to severe postsurgical complications.

Authors

Chapter 1

Esophageal Reconstruction with Large Intestine

1. Vascular anatomy of the colon

The colon is supplied with arterial blood from two main sources: the superior mesenteric artery (arteria mesenterica superior) and the inferior mesenteric artery (arteria mesenterica inferior). The right colon is supplied from the superior mesenteric artery through the following arteries: ileocolic artery (arteria ileo-colica), right colic artery (arteria colica dextra) and middle colic artery (arteria colica media). The inferior mesenteric artery supplies arterial blood to the left colon through the left colic artery (arteria colica sinistra). The ascending branch of the left colic artery (ramus ascendens) is joined with the middle colic artery by the arc of Riolan, creating in this way a connection between branches of inferior and superior mesenteric artery (Fig. 1, 2).

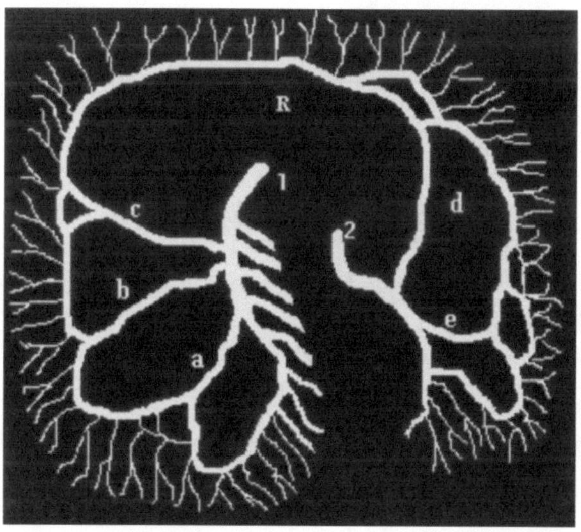

Figure 1 Diagram of the arterial blood supply to the colon: 1 –art. mesenterica superior, 2 – art. mesenterica inferior, a – art. ileocolica, b – art. colica dextra, c – art. colica media, d – ramus ascendens art. colicae sinistrae, e – ramus descendens art. colicae sinistrae, R – arcus Riolani

Individual vascular trunks of the right as well as of the left colon interconnect forming so-called arcades. The arc of Riolan, the longest vascular arcade, also known as the marginal artery, connects the blood vessels on the right and left part of the colon.

It is worth reminding that the ileocolic artery, the right colic artery and the left colic artery are situated behind the peritoneum, while the middle colic artery, arising from beneath the lower border of the pancreas, passes between the layers of the transverse mesocolon and directs to the hepatic flexure of the colon. Recollection of these well known anatomical facts is inasmuch significant as during preliminary intraoperative evaluation of the type of colon vasculature, it turns out that only mobilization of the ascending and the descending colon exposes clearly enough the topography of main vascular trunks and anastomoses between them, what in turn affects significantly the choice of adequately supplied and long colon segment for esophageal reconstruction. Topography of the venous drainage mirrors the arterial supply, i.e. arteries have respective vein equivalents.

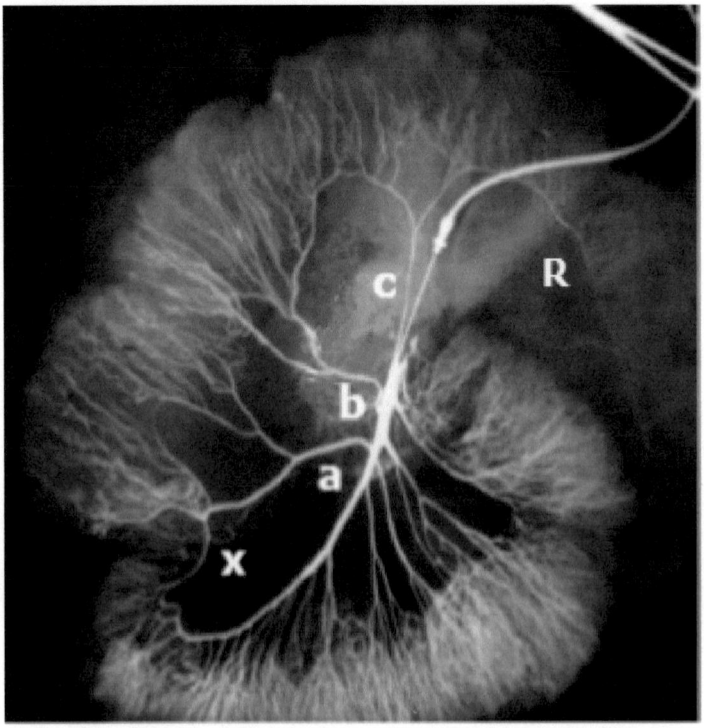

Figure 2 Angiogram of the superior mesenteric artery and its branches: X – the iliac branch of the ileocolic artery, a – art. ileocolica, b – art. colica dextra, c – art. colica media, R- arcus Riolani

The above vascular anatomy of the colon is what we can read in human anatomy textbooks. In clinical practice we meet certain deviations from the above presented topography. They usually concern the right colon and the venous system (Fig. 3).

Own experimental studies as well as studies by other authors on intestinal preparations demonstrate that 6% of population present with lack or hypoplasia of arcades anastomosing the main venous trunks with simultaneously well developed arterial trunks and broad and well developed arterial arcades within the right colon. In such cases the right colon cannot be used for reconstruction due to inadequate venous system. Angiographic evaluations of the colonic arterial system reveal that permanent arteries present in 100% of population include the ilecolic artery, the middle colic artery and the left colic artery. Well developed arc of Riolan is met in 90% of population, and about 50% have good anastomoses between all colic arteries. The right colic artery is absent in about 30-35% of population (Fig. 4). In 25% of population, its absence is compensated for by 1 to 3 so-called additional middle colic arteries. However the arteries are usually short, with a narrow lumen and the anastomosing arcades are also short and narrow.

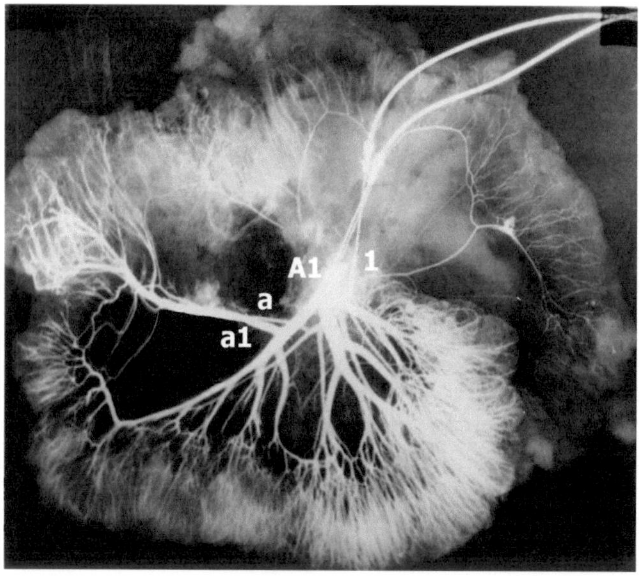

Figure 3 Angiogram of the superior mesenteric vessels: 1 – art. mesenterica superior, A1 – vena mesenterica superior, a – art. ileocolica, well developed, with efficient anastomosing arcades, a1 – vena ileocolica with bushy branches, does not form anastomosing arcades

The above presented anatomical details of the arterial and venous vasculature of the colon are very important, as they play a crucial role in the choice of an adequate, i.e. with good arterial supply and efficient venous drainage, intestinal segment to form a pedicled graft of the colon.

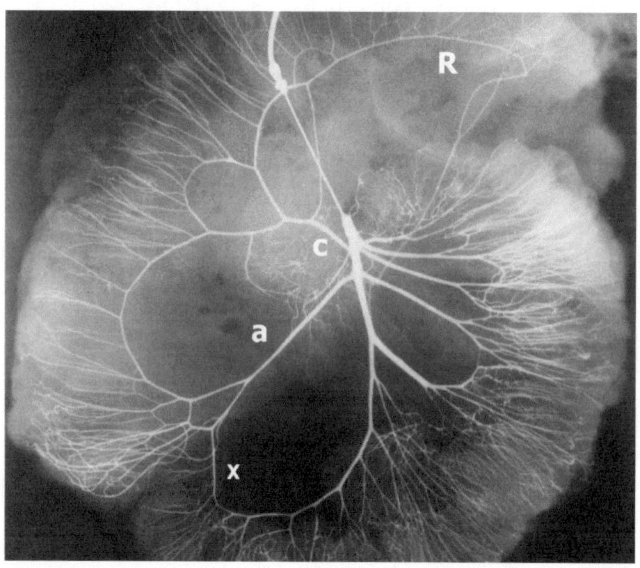

Figure 4 Angiogram of the superior mesenteric artery and its branches: X – the iliac branch of the ileocolic artery, a – art. ileocolica, c – art. colica media; absent art. colica dextra, R – arcus Riolani

2. Esophageal reconstructions using the colon

In order to organize and clarify descriptions of individual types of esophageal reconstructions, it should be remembered, as mentioned previously, that the main and at the same time permanent vessels of the colon include the ileocolic, middle colic and left colic vessels.

So-called adequate vascular systems in the aspect of reconstruction include long vascular trunks, which form wide arches passing into well developed and strong anastomosing arcades. The connection between the branches of the inferior and superior mesentery arteries, known as the arc of Riolan, is well developed. Such a situation gives the possibility of choosing either right, or left part of the colon to form a pedicled graft. For esophageal reconstruction each of the above mentioned colic vessels may be used to mobilize grafts in two positions: the isoperistaltic and the antiperistaltic grafts.

Selecting a segment of colon for esophageal reconstruction, one should always consider all the possibilities of the mobilization of the graft, in every individual case choosing the most suitable as far as blood supply and length is concerned pedicled segment of the colon. It should be remembered that the graft's length is strictly associated with the length of its vascular pedicle.

3. Esophageal reconstructions using the right colon

Taking advantage of an adequate vascular system in the colon, and choosing the right colon, the pedicled esophageal graft may be constructed using the following methods:

- from the right colon on ileocolic vascular pedicle in an antiperistaltic position of the graft
- from the right colon on middle colic vascular pedicle in an isoperistaltic position of the graft
- from the right colon on left colic vascular pedicle in an isoperistaltic position of the graft

3.1. The technique of creation of an antiperistaltic graft from the right colon on ileocolic vascular pedicle

The surgical technique presented below was developed by Prof. Jezioro in 1961 and used subsequently in the clinical practice in patients requiring esophageal reconstruction.

The abdominal cavity is approached from upper midline incision going several cm below and passing by the umbilicus on the right side. Next the right colon and the terminal segment of the ileum are mobilized. For this reason the small bowel loops are moved leftwards and maintained in this position with surgical towels. The parietal peritoneum is gradually transected starting from the iloecolic region next to the large bowel and continuing until the right flexure of the colon. Next, slightly elevating the bowel, the caecum and the ascending colon are separated together with blood vessels, and the ligaments of the right flexure of the colon are exposed and transected between ligatures. This maneuver allows to identify macroscopically and evaluate the structure and efficacy of the vascular system in this part of the colon in the aspect of esophageal reconstruction. The adequacy of circulation is ascertained when the arterial and venous trunks of the iloecolic vessels are long and well developed and the arcades anastomosing them to the right colon vessels, i.e. the right colic vessels and the latter and middle colic vessels are long and broad. If the right colic vessels are missing, they can be replaced by middle colic vessels. Next a biological trial is performed, i.e. the trunks of the right and middle colic vessels, iliac branch of the ileocolic vessels and the vascular arch between the middle colic vessels and the left colic vessels are clamped with vascular clamps, in order to create conditions resembling those in a graft pedicled exclusively on iloecolic vessels. The trial is considered positive when the separated intestinal segment maintains normal colour and reveals pulsation in the terminal intestinal vessels close to the intestinal wall. The evaluation of blood supply to the isolated intestinal segment may be confirmed by intraoperative ultrasound examination.

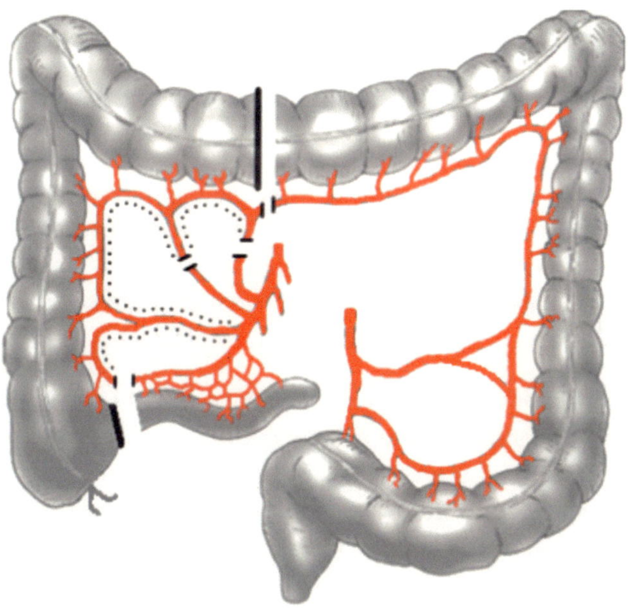

Figure 5 Diagram illustrating mobilization of a graft from the right colon on ileocolic vessels pedicle in an antiperistaltic position

Having evaluated the blood supply, with a positive outcome of the trial, the graft mobilization may start (Fig. 5, 6). The greater omentum is mobilized from the transverse colon to the middle of its length. Next the trunks of the right and middle colic vessels are ligated and transected. The transverse colon should be transected in the middle its length. The efferent transverse colon stump is sutured with a double-layer manual suture, or stapled. The vermiform appendix is excised in a routine manner. Subsequently, the iliac branch of the ileocolic vessels and terminal vessels of the caecal segment of the ileum are ligated and transected. The ileum is transected and the stumps are closed with a double-layer manual suture, or stapled. The caecal stump of the transected ileum should be short in order not to create a diverticular excess, what may have an unfavourable effect on subsequent function of the substitute esophagus.

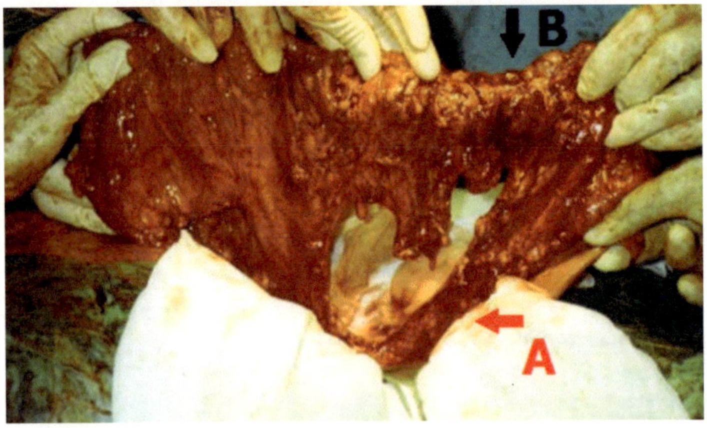

Figure 6 Intraoperative picture of mobilization of the right colon graft on ileocolic pedicle in an anti-peristaltic position. A –vascular pedicle, B – right colon

Cephalic stump of the graft, which is formed by the right transverse colon, is also closed with a double-layer manual suture, or stapled. In this way the stage of mobilization of the graft from the right colon on an ileocolic vascular pedicle is completed. Thus the reconstruction is antiperistaltic – the cephalic segment of the graft from the right colon will be anastomosed with the cervical esophagus, and the caecum – with the stomach.

The next stage includes construction of a retrosternal canal and passing the graft through a canal created in the interior mediastinum to the neck. Construction of the retrosternal canal requires special precision. This procedure should be initiated from the abdominal side in the following way. The xiphoid process of the sternum is exposed. Next the parietal peritoneum is separated from the diaphragm and the straight abdominal muscles and their origins are detached from the xiphoid process and the region of costal angles. Sharp retractors are placed onto the prepared costal arches and used to elevate the sternum (Fig. 7).

Preparing gently under visual control, and in close proximity to the posterior surface of the sternum, the pericardium and pleural layers should be mobilized to the level of mid-sternum. Then the canal should be widened to the sides and upwards to the neck, what requires special precision and carefulness. The canal is widened with the use of a metal spatula with a rounded tip, 3 cm wide and 30 cm long. Maneuvering gently the spatula under visual control, in close proximity to the posterior surface of the sternum, a wide retrosternal canal reaching the jugular notch of the episternum is constructed. Having completed the retrosternal canal from the abdominal side, the superior canal opening from the side of the neck should be formed.

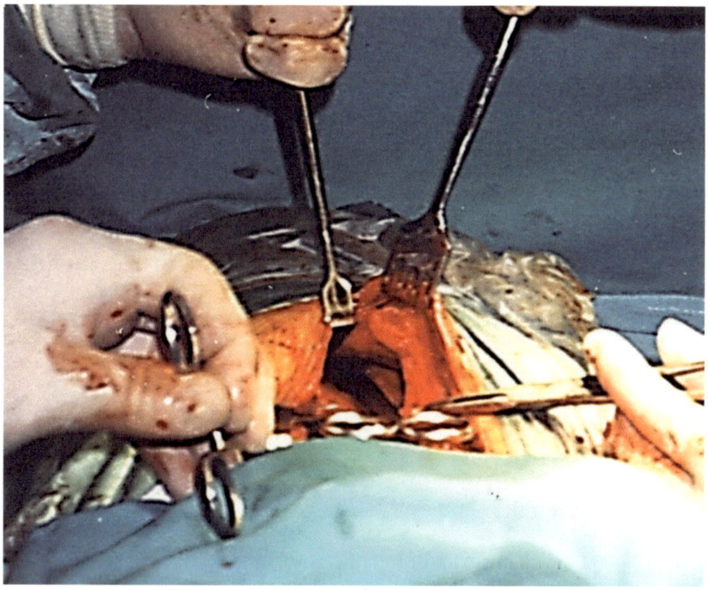

Figure 7 Intraoperative picture of retrosternal canal – image from the abdominal side

In case of patients with post-burn cicatrical stenosis of the thoracic esophagus, the cervical stage of the surgery is performed in the following way. The platysma muscle is exposed and transected with a skin incision on the left side of the neck, along and parallel to the anterior border of the sternocleidomastoid muscle, which is continued to the episternum. Next the left middle muscles of the neck (musculus sternothyreoideus et sternohyoideus) are exposed and transected at their sternal origin. In this way the left lobe of the thyroid gland is exposed. Further on, the loose connective tissue of the jugular fossa is dissected and, preparing gently along the lateral wall of the trachea, the anterior-medial border of the sternocleidomastoid muscle is exposed. The upper belly of the omohyoid muscle is transected at the level of the carotid artery triangle and the left superior and inferior thyroid vessels are mobilized. Ligature and transection of the superior and inferior thyroid vessels exposes the left-side wall of the pharynx and the cervical esophagus. When exposure of the pharynx is not necessary, it is enough to ligate and transect only the inferior thyroid vessels. Preparing gently in the tracheoesophageal sulcus below the larynx, the cervical esophagus is separated from the trachea. In order to facilitate the procedure, a rubber drain is placed onto the mobilized esophageal segment and, pulling slightly the drain, the whole cervical esophagus is exposed. Next traction sutures are placed in the lowest point of the cervical esophagus and the esophagus is transected transversely above the sutures. The distal stump of the esophagus supported on traction sutures is closed with a double-layer manual suture, or the whole procedure of transection and closure of the distal esophagus may be performed with the use of a surgical staple. The cervical esophagus, which is prepared for being anastomosed to the graft, is left covered with a sterile towel.

Next the retrosternal canal is opened from the side of the neck. The mediastinal adipose tissue should be dissected from the posterior surface of the sternum in the jugular fossa. Then, large cervical vessels and pleural laminae are carefully mobilized from the posterior sternum and the sternoclavicular joints, especially on the left, thus creating a sufficiently wide opening to the retrosternal canal from the side of the neck. Now a retractor is placed from the side of the neck on the mobilized episternum, and the sternum is gently pulled upwards. At the same time another retractor is placed on the xiphoid process from the side of the abdominal cavity. Elevating gently the sternum upwards and moving from the side of the neck and the abdomen, the retrosternal canal is widened on the sides, producing a canal that is wide enough on its whole length to hold the graft together with the vascular pedicle without tension.

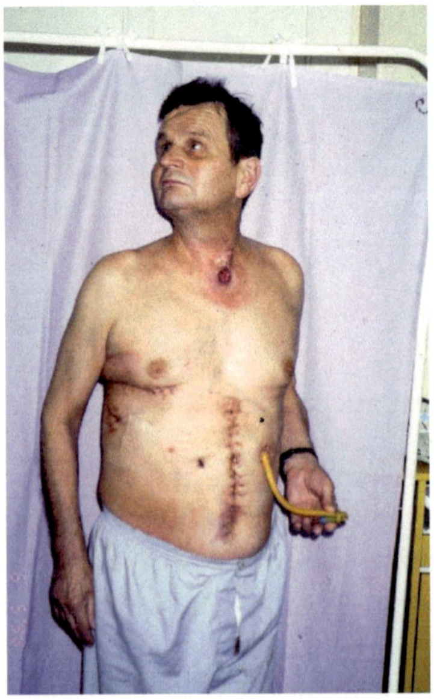

Figure 8 Picture of a patient after resection of thoracic oesophagus due to squamous cell oesophageal cancer (condition prior to oesophageal reconstruction).
on the neck – salivary fistula of the cervical esophagus;
on the right side of the chest – scar after thoracotomy;
in the epigastric midline – scar after laparotomy;
in the left hypochondrium – feeding gastric fistula

The next stage consists in placing the graft, which was formed during the abdominal stage of the operation, in the prepared retrosternal canal. For this reason, holding both previously placed retractors which elevate the sternum upwards, a thick long drain is inserted to the canal from the side of the neck, one arm of the drain leading from the canal to the epigastrium, the other being maintained on the neck. In order to shorten the graft's route, a colon segment mobilized on a vascular pedicle is passed beyond the stomach through an adequately wide slit, created in the hepatogastric ligament before it is placed in the retrosternal canal. The cephalic segment of the graft is fastened to the drain from the side of the abdomen. Gently pulling the drain's arm protruding from the side of the neck, the graft is pulled through the retrosternal canal and its cephalic part is exposed onto the neck in such a way as to enable its tensionless anastomosis to the cervical esophagus. Now the sternum-elevating retractors are removed. In this way the graft is positioned in the retrosternal canal. The part of the right colon which forms the cephalic segment of the graft is situated on the neck, while the caecum forming the caudal portion of the graft is anastomosed to the stomach. Thus constructed and placed in the retrosternal canal graft is arranged antiperistaltically. When the graft is left in the retrosternal canal, continuity of the gastrointestinal tract in the abdominal cavity should be restored, i.e. the ileum should be anastomosed to the distal part of the transverse colon. During this procedure the blood supply to the part of the graft emerging onto the neck should be monitored constantly. In case any features of ischemia appear in the graft segment emerging onto the neck, the graft must be immediately evacuated from the retrosternal canal and the cause of ischaemia removed. Only efficiently supplied graft authorizes its anastomosis to the cervical esophagus. Anastomosis of the caudal segment of the graft is performed in the prepyloric part of the stomach, what may prevent reflux of the gastric content to the replacement esophagus. Having performed all anastomoses within the abdominal cavity, the last stage of the reconstructive surgery may be performed – end-to-side anastomosis of the cervical esophagus with the lateral wall of the colon emerging onto the neck. The reconstructive surgery is finished when the abdominal integuments and the cervical integuments are closed.

In case of patients after resection of the thoracic esophagus due to cancer, the cervical stage of the surgery is slightly different than in individuals with post-burn cicatrical stenosis. In some patients resection of the thoracic portion of the esophagus due to cancer and reconstruction of the digestive tract continuity is performed in a single-stage operation. The excised esophagus is then replaced with the whole stomach, or a tube formed from the greater curvature of the stomach localized in the bed of the resected esophagus, i.e. in the posterior mediastinum. In patients, in whom single-stage esophageal reconstruction by means of stomach is not possible for various reasons, a reconstructive surgery with pedicled intestinal segment is considered. Due to a significant extent of the resection and reconstructive surgery, the procedure is performed in two stages. The first stage includes resection of the thoracic esophagus with lymphadenectomy, formation of a salivary fistula of the cervical esophagus, and a gastric or intestinal fistula for feeding the patient (Fig. 8). In the second stage, after several weeks, the retrosternal replacement esophagus is constructed with a pedicled colon segment. Mobilization of the pedicled colon segment, as well as creation of a retrosternal canal from the side of the abdomen is performed in the above-described manner, whereas opening of the retrosternal canal from the side of the neck is preceded by preparation of the salivary fistula and the cervical esophagus. The prepared segment of the cervical esophagus is covered with a surgical towel and placed on the upper border of the surgical wound on the neck. Opening of the retrosternal canal from the side of the neck is performed in the above-described way. When the retrosternal canal is wide enough from the side of the neck, as well as from the abdominal side, a mobilized pedicled colon segment is passed behind the sternum. Further procedures, i.e. restoration of the continuity of the gastrointestinal tract in the abdominal cavity, anastomosis of the caudal part of the graft with the stomach and anastomosis of the cephalic part of the graft with the cervical esophagus is performed in the same way as described in patients with post-burn cicatrical stenosis. In this group of patients the resection surgery is preceded by presurgical chemotherapy, or chemo- and radiotherapy. In some patients chemotherapy is administered as adjuvant therapy after resection of the esophagus and prior to reconstructive surgery. As the aim of the authors was to present only esophageal reconstructions with the use of pedicled intestinal segments, treatment of esophageal carcinoma will not be discussed in details.

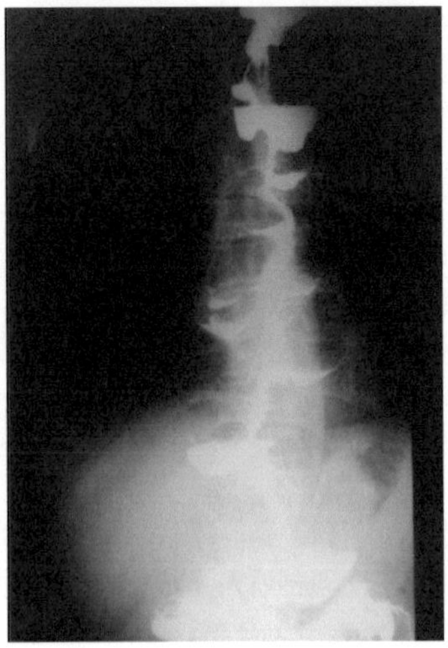

Figure 9 Radiogram of a replacement retrosternal oesophagus from the right colon on ileocolic vascular pedicle in an antiperistaltic position according to Jezioro

The above described modality of esophageal reconstruction is advantageous for a number of reasons. The operation is fairly simple technically, provided the vascular system in this part of the colon was evaluated accurately. Mobilization of the graft causes relatively small deficit of the intestine in the abdominal cavity. The graft, constructed according to the above-described method, is long enough, and may be anastomosed to the pharynx, for example in patients with obstructed cervical esophagus.

Theoretically, the only disadvantage of the reconstruction modality may be associated with an antiperistaltic position of the graft, although control studies in patients with antiperistaltic reconstructions did not confirm these fears (Fig. 9).

3.2. The technique of construction of an isoperistaltic graft from the right colon on middle colic vascular pedicle

The right colon may be also used to isolate another kind – an isoperistaltic colon graft pedicled on the middle colic artery. This type of graft is conditioned by the presence of well developed, long main vascular trunks within the right colon, which are anastomosed with broad, well developed and efficient arcades. The surgical modality presents as follows.

The abdominal cavity is opened through an upper midline incision passing by the umbilicus and going 2-3 cm below. The next stage is to mobilize the right colon and the terminal segment of the ileum in a manner presented above, what enables macroscopic evaluation of the vascular system in this part of the colon. On finding a positive vascular structure, a biological trial should be performed, in which the trunks of the ileocolic and right colic vessels are clamped with vascular clamps, thus leaving the selected part of the colon supplied only by the middle colic vessels. It should be remembered that in some patients the right colic vessels are missing (see: Fig. 4), and the middle colic vessels are shaped in the form of two or three additional colic vessels. In such cases, with narrow arcades joining the middle colic vessels and the additional middle colic vessels, the use of both middle colic trunks as the graft pedicle may be considered, provided the double pedicle does not shorten the length of the mobilized colon graft. Any disturbances in the blood supply to the graft, arterial or venous, observed during the biological trial, oblige to resign from this part of the colon and impose selection of another, adequately supplied, segment of the large intestine.

In case the result of the biological trial is positive and no disturbances in the blood supply to the isolated fragment of the colon are observed, mobilization of the graft may be initiated. First the greater omentum is removed in the area of the mobilized colon segment, and next the vascular trunks, which had been clamped in vascular clamps, are ligated and transected. In some cases the arterial trunk should be ligated separately from the venous trunk, as they are often distant and their jointly ligation may contribute to shortening of the vascular pedicle in the mobilized graft. Next the transverse colon should be transected in the middle of its length. The efferent stump of the transverse colon is closed with a double-layer manual suture, or stapled. On the other hand, the afferent stump, which forms the caudal segment of the mobilized graft, is closed with a temporary suture until it is anastomosed with the stomach. Transection of the ileum in the caecal region completes mobilization of the graft. The stumps of the transected ileum are closed with a double-layer manual suture, or stapled, close to the caecum, without leaving diverticular excess. Appendectomy is performed in a routine manner. The isoperistaltic graft from the right colon pedicled on the middle colic artery is thus constructed (Fig. 10).

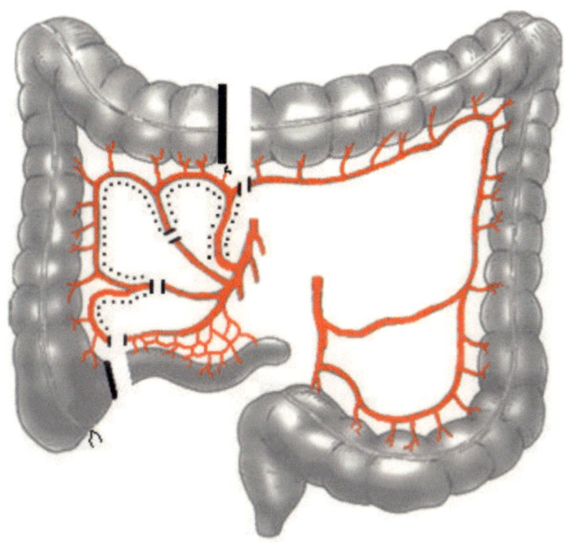

Figure 10 Diagram of mobilization of a right colon graft together with the caecum on middle colic vascular pedicle in an isoperistaltic position

Further steps are similar to those presented above. They include construction of the retrosternal canal, placement of the graft in the canal, restoration of gastrointestinal continuity and anastomosing the graft with the stomach and the cervical esophagus.

The above-presented modality of esophageal reconstruction has many advantages. At the same time it is not free from certain disadvantages. The most significant advantages include an isoperistaltic position of the graft, what undoubtedly has a positive effect on its functioning as an esophageal replacement. Making a decision as to the choice of the above described reconstructive modality, it should be remembered that it is conditioned by the presence of an exceptionally effective vascular system within the right colon. In case additional middle colic vessels are present, they usually have relatively short trunks, and shorter and narrower anastomosing arcades, and for these reasons the mobilized graft may turn out to be too short to be anastomosed to the cervical esophagus. Another disadvantage is a large mass of the cephalic segment of the graft, i.e. the caecum, what may hamper safe passage of the graft through the superior opening of the retrosternal canal just beyond the left sternoclavicular joint. Pressure present in the region of the superior opening of the canal leads to irreversible ischemic changes and severe postsurgical complications, in form of necrosis of the cephalic segment of the graft. In order to prevent such complications, it is necessary to perform partial or complete removal of the joint, what is practiced in some surgical centres.

In cases, in which very long main vascular trunks in the right colon are found during the operation, and the anastomosing arcades are also long and wide, a similar graft may be constructed, but without participation of the caecum. Then slightly longer segment of the transverse colon should be mobilized. Such a variant of operation is possible when, apart from an adequate vascular system in the right colon, also the arc of Riolan is very well developed. In this way problems associated with the presence of the caecum, which forms the cephalic portion of the graft, may be avoided in some cases. Choosing this surgical modality, we obtain an isoperistaltic graft with a straight shape and significantly narrower diameter in the cephalic portion (Fig. 11).

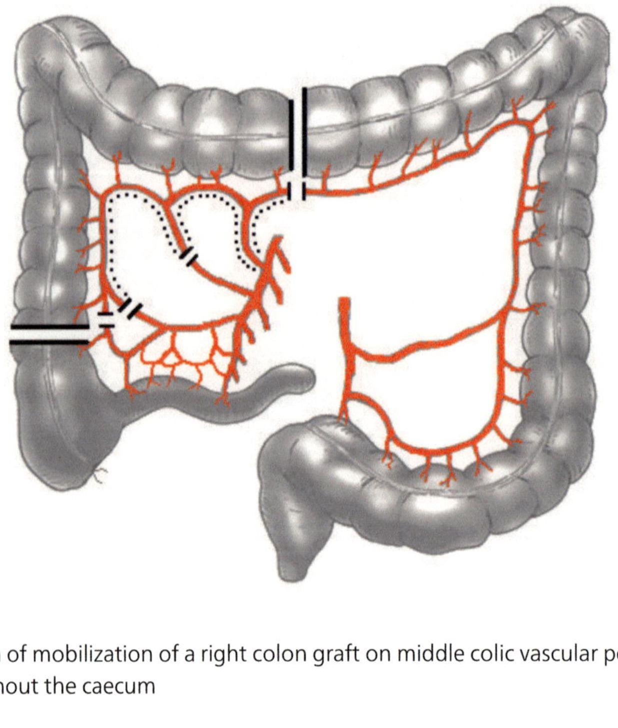

Figure 11 Diagram of mobilization of a right colon graft on middle colic vascular pedicle in an isoperistaltic position without the caecum

As it was described in the previous section, the next stage of the operation includes construction of the retrosternal canal and passage of the graft through the canal created in the anterior mediastinum. In order to obtain sufficient mobility of the graft, it is worth considering reducing the caudal portion of the intestinal segment which will be anastomosed to the stomach. The graft is then passed behind the stomach through a hole formed in the hepatogastric ligament and placed in the created retrosternal canal. The proximal segment of the graft, i.e. the caecum is exposed onto the neck, if the first variant of the reconstructive surgery was chosen. If mobilization of the graft was done according to the second variant, i.e. without participation of the caecum, the ascending colon is exposed on the neck. Anastomoses within the abdominal cavity restoring the gastrointestinal continuity as well as anastomosis of the caudal portion of the graft with the anterior wall of the prepyloric part of the stomach complete the abdominal stage of the reconstructive surgery. The last stage includes anastomosing the cervical esophagus to the lateral wall of the colon exposed to the neck. Suturing of the abdominal layers and the neck terminates the reconstructive surgery.

Remote follow up examinations in patients after reconstructive surgery performed according to the above described modality revealed efficient function of the replacement esophagus (Fig. 12, 13).

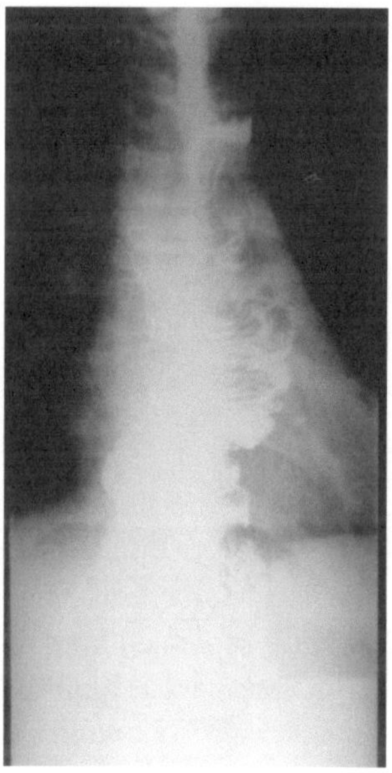

Figure 12 Radiogram of a replacement retrosternal oesophagus from the right colon on middle colic vascular pedicle in an isoperistaltic position. A-P projection

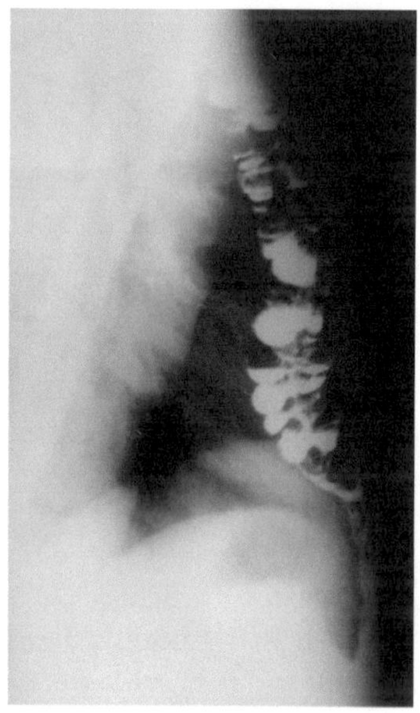

Figure 13 Radiogram of a replacement retrosternal oesophagus from the right colon on middle colic vascular pedicle in an isoperistaltic position. Lateral projection

3.3. The technique of construction of an isoperistaltic graft from the right colon on left colic vascular pedicle

Construction of a graft pedicled on the left colic artery is another possibility of using the right colon for esophageal reconstruction. This variant of the reconstructive surgery is much more complicated and requires excellent surgical technique as well as careful intraoperative evaluation of the colonic vasculature. This surgical modality may be used only when the right colonic as well as the left colonic circulation is highly adequate and the arc of Riolan is very well developed. The main advantage of this surgical modality is the possibility of obtaining a very long graft. The risks however concern the vascular pedicle. The graft is supplied from the left colic vessels, but the only, very long, route of blood supply to the whole graft is from the arc of Riolan. With an erroneous evaluation of the efficacy of the graft vasculature, this situation may lead to peripheral ischaemia of the mobilized segment of the colon. For this reason, when a decision is made to choose this reconstructive modality, the intraoperative biological trial of vascular efficiency should be meticulously performed and accurately evaluated.

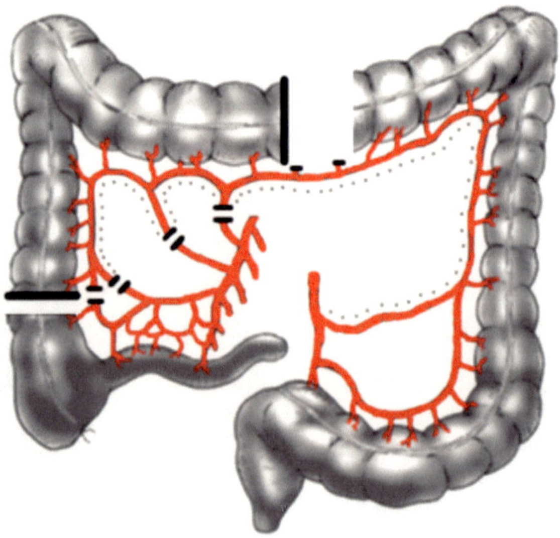

Figure 14 Diagram of mobilization of a right colon graft on left colic vascular pedicle in an isoperistaltic position

Technically this modality is much more difficult than those previously described. After laparotomy it is necessary to mobilize the right colon. The greater omentum is separated from the transverse colon on its whole length. The result of the biological trial plays a decisive role. If, after clamping the trunks of the middle and right colic vessels and the arch joining the ileocolic vessels and the right colic vessels, the observed colon does not reveal any signs of ischaemia, further mobilization of the colonic segment may proceed. The left flexure of the colon and the descending colon should be mobilized. For this reason the small intestine loops are moved to the right side of the abdominal cavity and maintained in this position with surgical towels. The peritoneum is transected longitudinally on the external side of the descending colon as well as on the right side. Next, slightly elevating the colon, the descending colon is carefully separated together with its vessels and the left flexure of the colon is exposed. Ligaments supporting the flexure are cut between ligatures.

In the next stage of the surgery the vessels trunks which were previously clamped, i.e. the right colic, middle colic and the arches between the right colic and ileocolic vessels are ligated and transected. Also the ascending colon is transected at this level. Remembering that the graft has to be long enough to reach the neck where it is anastomosed to the cervical esophagus, a longer or shorter segment of the transverse colon is selected and cut at this level. Reduction performed in the caudal portion of the graft permits to achieve its adequate mobility, and free from tension in the vascular pedicle translocation of thus mobilized graft beyond the stomach, and next, through the retrosternal canal, onto the neck (Fig. 14). Subsequently the continuity of the gastrointestinal tract in the abdominal cavity should be restored and the caudal portion of the graft should be anastomosed to the stomach. The reconstructive surgery is complete when the cephalic segment of the graft is anastomosed to the cervical esophagus.

The advantageous points of this reconstructive modality include the possibility of obtaining the longest graft of all previously described variants using the right colon provided the above conditions concerning blood supply to the mobilized graft are fulfilled. Another advantage of the presented modality is the isoperistaltic position of the graft, what has a beneficial effect on its further functioning as a replacement esophagus (Fig. 15, 16). The only disadvantage is theoretically much more difficult surgical technique in comparison to previously described variants.

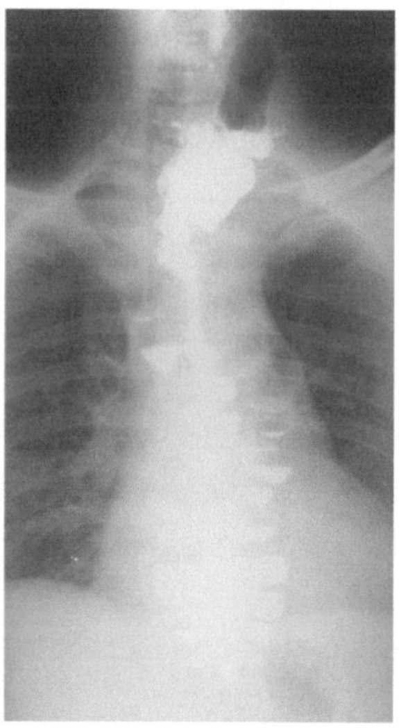

Figure 15 Radiogram of a replacement retrosternal oesophagus from the right colon on left colic vascular pedicle in an isoperistaltic position. A-P projection

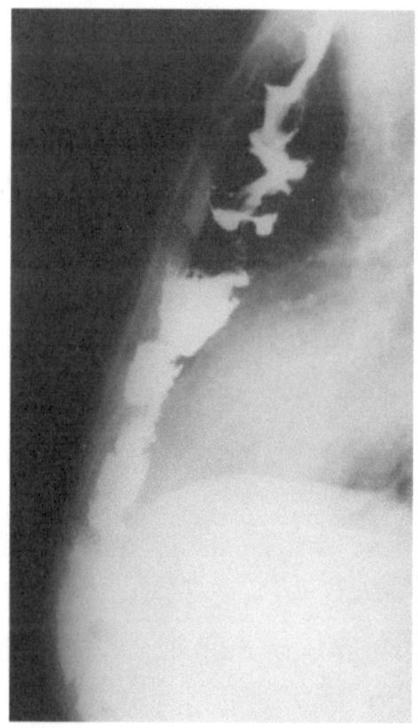

Figure 16 Radiogram of a replacement retrosternal oesophagus from the right colon on left colic vascular pedicle in an isoperistaltic position. Lateral projection

4. Esophageal reconstructions using the left colon

The presence of advantageous vasculature systems in the right and left halves of the colon as well as efficient arc of Riolan provide opportunities of using the left colon to create a pedicled esophageal graft in the following ways:

- from the left colon on the middle colic vascular pedicle in an antiperistaltic position of the graft

- from the left colon on the left colic vascular pedicle in an isoperistaltic position of the graft
- from the left colon on the left colic vascular pedicle in an antiperistaltic position of the graft

4.1. The technique of construction of an antiperistaltic graft from the left colon on middle colic vascular pedicle

An adequate vascular system in the left colon as well as well developed arc of Riolan provide an opportunity to use this segment of colon to construct an antiperistaltic graft pedicled on middle colic vessels.

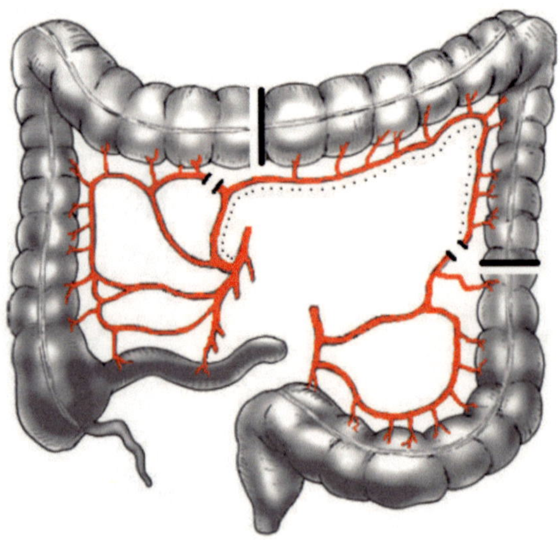

Figure 17 Diagram of mobilization of a left colon graft on middle colic vascular pedicle in an antiperistaltic position

The surgical technique is as follows. The abdominal cavity is opened through the upper midline incision passing by the umbilicus. Next the left colon is mobilized and the biological trial of vascular efficiency is performed. For this reason ligaments of the left flexure of the colon are transected. The left colon together with its vasculature is separated from the posterior abdominal wall as far as the site where the left colic vessels branch off the main trunk of the inferior mesenteric vessels. Next the greater omentum is isolated and the biological trial is performed. The ascending branch of the left colic vessels are clamped with hemostatic forceps nearby ramification of the main trunk into the ascending and the descending branches. Next clamp forceps are applied on the arch between the middle colic and right colic vessels. If the blood supply to the colon is unaffected, mobilization of the graft from the left colon on middle colic vessels may proceed (Fig. 17). The previously clamped vessels should be ligated and transected. In order to obtain a straight graft, the transverse mesocolon is incised radially, terminating the incision 2-3 cm away from the arc of Riolan. The transverse colon is transected beyond the ramification of the middle colic vessels. The afferent stump of the transverse colon is closed tight, and the efferent stump, which will form the caudal part of the graft, and will be anastomosed to the stomach, is closed with temporary sutures. In order to determine situationally the site of transection of the descending colon, it should be remembered that the length of graft is the length of its vascular pedicle. The length of the pedicle may be measured approximately using a long thread which measures the length from the stomach angle to the angle of the mandible on the left side of the neck. When the needed length of the pedicle is approximated in this way, the same thread may be used to determine the site of transection of the descending colon by measuring the distance from the region of the middle colic vessels trunk, and, further on, along the arc of Riolan and along the ascending branch of the left colic vessels. Both stumps of the transected descending colon are closed tight with manual sutures, or stapled. The proximal stump of the descending colon will create the cephalic part of the graft. Thus the left colon graft pedicled on the middle colic vessels is constructed. The graft will be in antiperistaltic position.

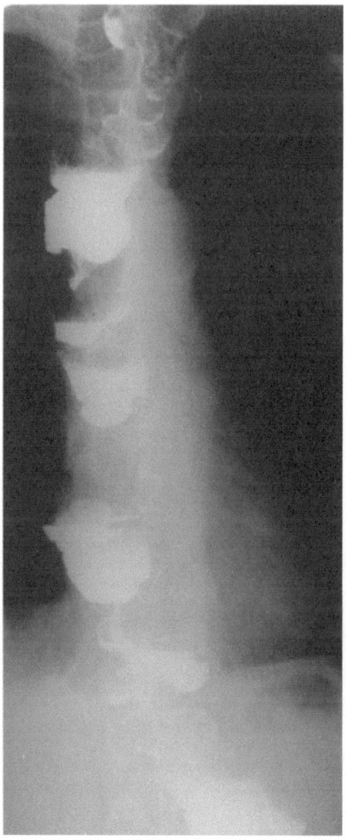

Figure 18 Radiogram of a replacement retrosternal oesophagus from the left colon on middle colic vascular pedicle in an antiperistaltic position. A-P projection

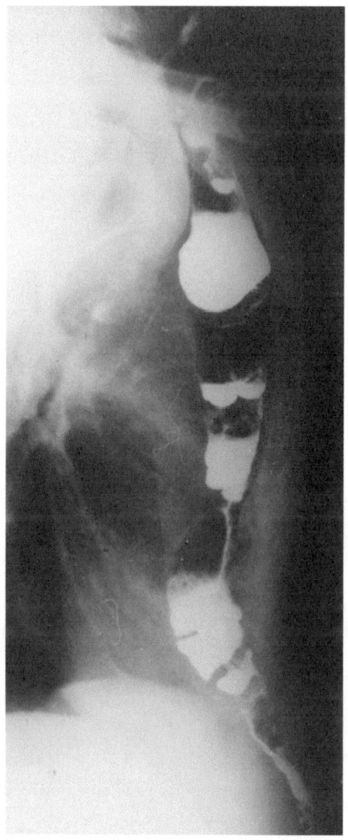

Figure 19 Radiogram of a replacement retrosternal oesophagus from the left colon on middle colic vascular pedicle in an antiperistaltic position. Lateral projection

Having constructed the retrosternal canal in a mode described previously, the graft is passed beyond the stomach and through the canal. The descending colon is exposed on the neck, and distal, caudal part of the graft, formed by the transverse colon, remains in the abdominal cavity to be anastomosed to the stomach. For safe, tensionless restoration of the continuity of the gastrointestinal tract, the hepatic flexure of the colon is mobilized and the colon stumps remaining after mobilization of the graft are anastomosed. Anastomosis of the distal, caudal part of the graft to the stomach terminates the reconstructive surgery. The last stage includes anastomosis of the esophagus with the colon pulled onto the neck. Using the end-to-side anastomosis of the esophagus with the lateral wall of the colon, the anastomosis lumen is wide enough to have a beneficial effect on the function of the antiperistaltic esophageal reconstruction (Fig. 18, 19).

The main advantage of this surgical modality is a relatively simple surgical technique, provided the adequacy of circulation has been evaluated accurately. On the other hand, antiperistaltic position of the graft may be its less advantageous feature, which may slow down the passage of the content through the replacement esophagus.

4.2. The technique of construction of an isoperistaltic graft from the left colon on left colic vascular pedicle

Taking advantage of adequate vasculature in the left colon, finding a long trunk of the left colic vessels, the arc of Riolan and the presence of long, well developed anastomoses between the left colic vessels and sigmoid vessels an isoperistaltic graft with left colic vascular pedicle may be constructed.

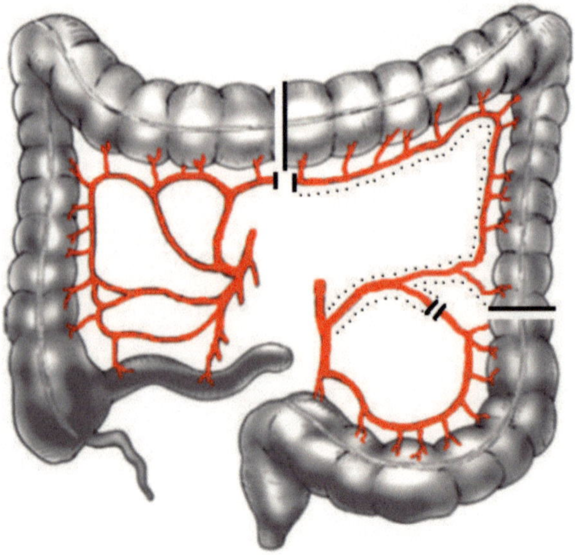

Figure 20 Diagram of mobilization of a left colon graft on left colic vascular pedicle in an isoperistaltic position

The applied technique is as follows. The abdominal cavity is opened in a routine manner through an upper midline incision passing by the umbilicus. Thorough evaluation of topography of the left colon vasculature may be performed after its full mobilization and separation of the greater omentum. If the macroscopic picture of vasculature presents favourably in the aspect of graft mobilization, a meticulous trial of the efficiency of the left colic vessels should be performed. The arch joining the middle colic vessels and the left colic vessels as well as the arch joining the left colic vessels and the sigmoid vessels are clamped with hemostatic forceps. In this way the arterial blood supply and the venous blood flow in the left part of the colon are carried out trough the left colic vessels alone. A positive biological trial entitles to mobilize the graft. The previously clamped arch of the middle colic vessels should be ligated and transected close to the ramification of the main trunk. The transverse mesocolon should be incised radially, what straightens the graft and facilitates its further mobilization. Next the vascular arch joining the left colic vessels with the sigmoid vessels, the transverse colon, and the descending colon are ligated and transected. The stumps of the transected colon are closed tight by means of a surgical stapler, or a manual suture. In this way an isoperistaltic graft from the left colon on left colic vessels pedicle is mobilized (Fig. 20).

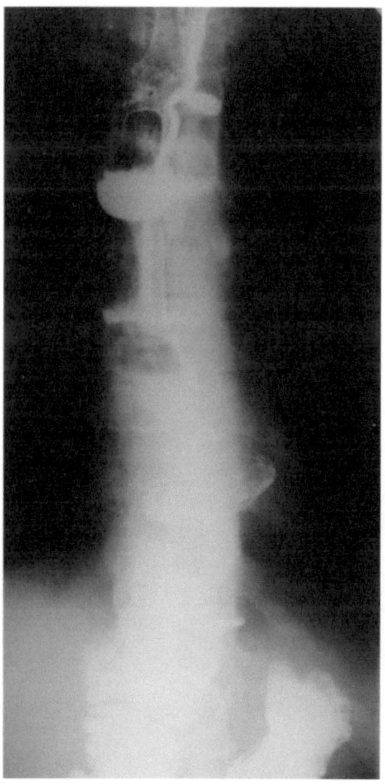

Figure 21 Radiogram of a replacement retrosternal oesophagus from the left colon on left colic vascular pedicle in an isoperistaltic position. A-P projection

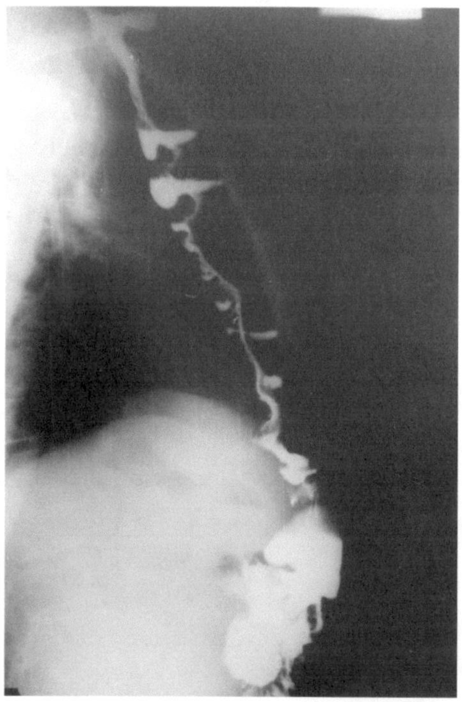

Figure 22 Radiogram of a replacement retrosternal oesophagus from the left colon on left colic vascular pedicle in an isoperistaltic position. Lateral projection

Subsequently the graft is passed beyond the stomach and placed in the retrosternal canal. The proximal part of the graft, i.e. the transverse colon creates the cephalic part of the replacement esophagus will be anastomosed to the cervical esophagus. The last stage of the reconstructive abdominal surgery includes anastomosing the remaining proximal colon with distal part of the sigmoid colon and the caudal part of the graft with the anterior wall of the prepyloric stomach. Cervical anastomosis and closing the neck and abdominal layers is the last stage of the whole reconstructive surgery.

Advantages of this modality include isoperistaltic position of the graft, its straight course in the retrosternal canal, as well as definitely narrower lumen in comparison to the grafts formed from the right colon (Fig. 21, 22).

The fact that in some cases the trunk of the left colic vessels may be well developed, but turns out to be too short to produce a long enough graft which would reach the neck is a disadvantage of this type of reconstructive surgery.

4.3. The technique of construction of an antiperistaltic graft from the left colon on left colic vascular pedicle

Choosing this modality to construct a pedicled graft, the architecture of vasculature in the left colon and proximal sigmoid colon must be evaluated exceptionally meticulously, as this method is possible only in such cases in which the main trunk of left colic vessels (arteries and veins) is very long, the descending branch is well developed, exceptionally long, and at the same time it creates firm and efficient anastomoses with the sigmoid vessels.

The surgical technique resembles this described in the previous chapter. The differences include an antiperistaltic position of the graft and the left colic vessels pedicle. Thus in order to obtain an adequately long graft, it is almost always necessary to use the left colon with a proximal segment of the sigmoid colon. Accurate evaluation of the length of the vascular pedicle is decisive for success in obtaining such a graft.

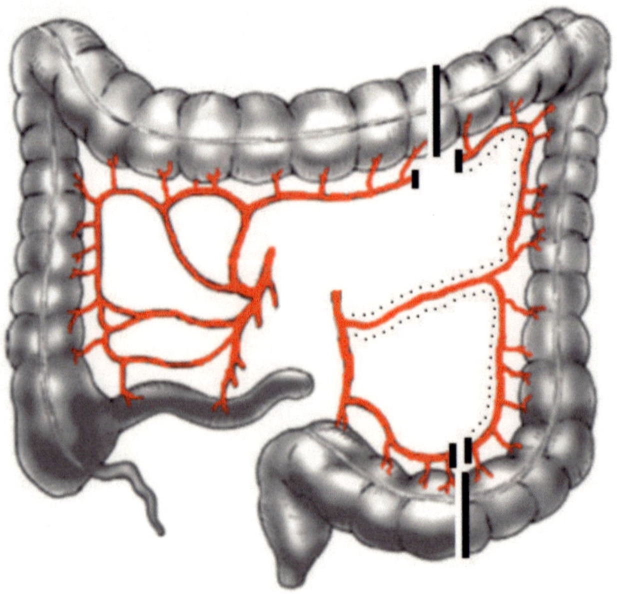

Figure 23 Diagram of mobilization of a left colon graft on left colic vascular pedicle in an antiperistaltic position

If the vascular system is considered adequate, the left colon should be mobilized and a thorough intraoperative biological trial of vascular efficiency should be performed in order to confirm once again pertinence of the choice. Full mobilization of the graft takes place after ligation and transection at an adequate level of the ascending branch and the descending branch of the left colic artery and vein, and next of the transverse colon and the sigmoid colon (Fig. 23). Thus constructed graft will be antiperistaltic, that is its distal, caudal part, i.e. the descending colon or proximal segment of the sigmoid colon will be anastomosed to the cervical esophagus, while the proximal part, i.e. the transverse colon – to the anterior wall of the prepyloric part of the stomach.

Subsequent stages of the procedure, as described previously, consist in restoring the continuity of the gastrointestinal tract in the abdominal cavity and anastomosing the pedicled colon segment, which was passed through the retrosternal canal, to the cervical esophagus and the stomach.

The surgical technique of this reconstructive modality is not easy. This especially concerns an accurate evaluation of the length of the vascular pedicle. This type of esophageal reconstruction should be reserved to exceptional cases – with inadequate vascular system in the right colon, precluding reconstruction by means of another and easier method. Moreover, it is not recommended for surgeons with little experience in reconstructive procedures. Antiperistaltic position of the graft may also be considered disadvantageous. Advantages of this surgical modality include the graft's straight course in the retrosternal canal, as well as a definitely narrower lumen in comparison to right colon grafts (Fig. 24).

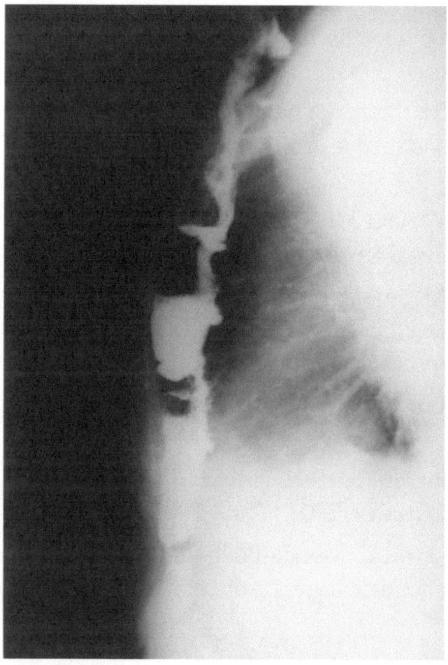

Figure 24 Radiogram of a replacement retrosternal oesophagus from the left colon on left colic vascular pedicle in an antiperistaltic position. Lateral projection.

Presenting the above described esophageal reconstructions with the colon, important technical details as well as modes of choosing individual reconstructive modality with the use of right or left colon were described. Also, advantages and disadvantages of individual modalities were presented, taking into account functions the replacement esophagus has to perform.

5. References

[1] Kelling G. Ösophagoplastik mit hilfe des querkolon. Zentralbl Chir 1911, 36: 1209-1213.

[2] Vulliet H. De l'oesophagoplastieet des diverses modifications. Semaine Med 1911, 31: 529-530.

[3] Rauber-Kopsch F. Lehrbbuch und Atlas der Anatomie des Menschen. Abteilung 3, Ed Leipzig, Georg Thiema, 1923, 321-393.

[4] Sonneland J, Anson BJ, Beaton LE. Surgical anatomy of the arterial supply to the colon from the superior mesenteric artery based upon a study of 600 specimens. Surg Gynecol Obstet 1958, 106: 385-398.

[5] Schumacher GH. Human topographic anatomy. Ed 1, Volumed, Wrocław, Poland, 1994, p 259-261.

[6] Popovici Z. Angiographic research on the blood supply of the colon with a view to oesophagoplasty. J Chir 1977, 113, 517-526.

[7] Jezioro Z, Milnerowicz S. Classification of reconstructive surgery of the whole esophagus using the large intestine and based on angiographic studies. Pol Przegl Chir 1978, 50: 461-465.

[8] Cheng BC. Clinical study of colic vessels with respect to their significance in the replacement of the esophagus by the colon. Zhonghua Wai Ke Za Zhi 1989, 27: 566-568, 575-576.

[9] Makuuchi H. Reconstruction after thoracic esophagectomy. Nihon Geka Gakkai Zasshi 2008, 109: 256-260.

[10] Strutyńska-Karpińska M. Causes of blood perfusion disturbances in pedunculated intestinal grafts employed in reconstructive procedures of the esophagus. Pol Przegl Chir 1993, 65: 1185-1190.

[11] Peters JH, Kronson JW, Katz M, DeMester TR. Arterial anatomic considerations in colon interposition for esophageal replacement. Arch Surg 1995, 130: 858-862.

[12] Strutyńska-Karpińska M. Studies on the vascularization of the ileum and the right half of the colon in view of the possibilities of employing the above intestinal segments in reconstructive operations of the entire esophagus. Pol Przegl Chir 1995, 67: 1204-1213.

[13] Lorenzini L, Bertelli L, Lorenzi M. Arterial supply in the left colonic flexure. Ann Ital Chir 1999, 70: 691-698.

[14] Predescu D, Constantinoiu S. Problems and difficulties in patients with esophageal reconstruction. Chirugia (Bucur) 2002, 97:187-201.

[15] Chirica M, de Chaisemartin C, Munoz-Bongrand N, Halimi B, Celerier M, Cattan P, Sarfati E. Colonic interposition for esophageal replacement after caustic ingestion. J Chir (Paris) 2009, 146: 240-249.

[16] Nguyen DH, Pham TA, Nguyen CM. Anterothoracic colonic replacement in cicatricial caustic strictures of the esophagus in a 1-stage procedure. Zentralbl Chir, 1984, 109:472-478.

[17] Ngan SYK, Wong J. Lengths of different routes for esophageal replacement. J Thorac Cardiovasc Surg 1986, 91: 790-792.

[18] Rakić S, Diuranović S. Lengths of different routes for esophageal replacement in a white population. J Thorac Cardiovasc Surg 1993, 105: 1122.

[19] Strutyńska-Karpińska M. Retrosternal canal in reconstructive procedures of the entire esophagus. Pol Przegl Chir 1997, 69: 1191-1196.

[20] Nienartowicz M, Nienartowicz E, Grabowski K, Strutyńska-Karpińska M, Błaszczuk J, Szelachowski P. Preoperative evaluation of the upper section of the retrosternal tunnel in esophageal reconstruction procedures. Adv Clin Exp Med 2009, 18: 159-162.

[21] Hu H, Ye T, Tan D, Li H, Chen H. Is anterior mediastinum route a shorter choice for esophageal reconstruction? A comparative anatomic study. Eur J Cardiothorac Surg 2011, 40:1466-1469.

[22] Lafargue P, Dufour R, Cabanie H, Chavannaz J. Prethoracic esophagoplasty using the right colon and the terminal ileum. Mem Acad Chir 1951, 77: 362-372.

[23] Scanlon EF, Staley CJ. The use of the ascending and right half of the transverse colon in esophagoplasty. Surg Gynecol Obstet 1958, 107: 99-103.

[24] Jezioro Z. Antiperistaltic esophagoplasty using the right half of the colon. Zentralbl Chir 1961, 86: 1739-1744.

[25] Hong PW, Seel D, Dietrick RB. The use of colon in repair of benign stricture of the esophagus. Pac Med Surg 1967, 75: 148-155.

[26] Negre E, Coulon P. Presternal ileum and right colon for benign esophageal stenosis. Very long-term checking. J Chir (Paris) 1984, 121: 639-642.

[27] El-Domeiri A, Martini N, Beattie EJ. Esophageal reconstruction by colon interposition. Arch Surg 1970, 100: 358-362.

[28] Ventemiglia R, Khalil KG, Frazier OH, Mountain CF. The role of preoperative mesenteric arteriography in colon interposition. J Thorac Cardiovasc Surg 1977, 74: 98-108.

[29] Nicks R. Colonic replacement of the oesophagus. Br J Surg 1967, 54: 124-128.

[30] Fürst H, Hartl WH, Löhe F, Schildberg FW. Colon interposition for esophageal replacement: an alternative technique based on the use of the right colon. Ann Surg 2000, 231: 173-178.

[31] Fürst H, Hartl WH, Löhe F, Schildberg FW. German experience with colon interposition grafting as an esophageal substitute. Dis Esophagus 2001, 14: 131-134.

[32] Strutynska-Karpinska M. Oesophageal reconstruction with right part of colon. Adv Clin Exp Med 2004, 13:151-161.

[33] Bothereau H, Munoz-Bongrand N, Lambert B, Montemagno S, Cattan P, Sarfati E. Esophageal reconstruction after caustic injury: is there still a place for right coloplasty? Am J Surg 2007, 193: 660-664.

[34] Thomas P, Giudicelli R, Fuentes P, Reboud E. Technique and results of colonic esophagoplasties. Ann Chir 1996, 50: 106-120.

[35] Mutaf O, Avanoglu A. Oesophagoplasty in the treatment of caustic oesophageal strictures in children. Br J Surg 1995, 82: 644-646.

[36] Young MM, Deschamps C, Trastek VF, Allen MS, Miller DL, Schleck CD, Pailorelo PC. Esophageal reconstruction for benign disease: Early morbidity, mortality, and functional results. Ann Thorac Surg 2000, 70: 1651-1655.

[37] Orsoni P, Toupet A. Use of the descending colon and the left part of the transverse colon for prethoracic esophagoplasty. Presse Med 1950, 58: 804-806.

[38] Strutynska-Karpinska M. Oesophageal reconstruction with left part of colon. Adv Clin Exp Med 2004, 13:163-169.

[39] Montenegro EB, Cutait DE, Ramos de Oliveira M, Fanganiello M, Faria SG, Morgante PA. Transthoracic esophagoplasty for benign stricture by means of transverse colon. Surg 1953, 34: 313-318.

[40] Stephens HB. Colon bypass of the esophagus. Am J Surg 1971, 122: 217-222.

[41] Gregorie HB Jr. Esophagocoloplasty. Ann Surg 1972, 175: 740-751.

[42] Chien KY, Wang PY, Lu KS. Esophagoplasty for corrosive stricture of the esophagus: an analysis of 60 cases. Ann Surg 1974, 179: 510-515.

[43] Wilkins EW, Burke JF. Colon esophageal bypass. Am J Surg 1975, 129: 394-400.

[44] Belsey RHR. Palliative management of esophageal carcinoma. Am J Surg 1980, 139: 789-794.

[45] Mansour KA, Hansen HA, Hersh T, Miller JI, Hatcher CR. Colon interposition for advanced nonmalignant esophageal stricture: experience with 40 patients. Ann Thorac Surg 1981, 32: 584-591.

[46] Postlethwait RW. Colonic interposition for esophageal substitution. Surg Gynecol Obstet 1983, 156: 377-383.

[47] Ribet M, Barrat C. Colonic esophagoplasty for benign lesions. Ann Chir 1995, 49: 133-137.

[48] Knezević JD, Radovanović NS, Simić AP, Kotarac MM, Skrobić OM, Konstantinović VD, Pesk PM. Colon interposition in the treatment of esophageal caustic strictures: 40 years of experience. Dis Esophagus 2007, 20: 530-534.

[49] Strutyńska-Karpińska M. Early postoperative complications in reconstructive operations of the esophagus. Pol Przegl Chir 1997, 69: 677-685.

[50] Milnerowicz S, Grabowski K, Strutyńska-Karpińska M, Knast W. Gastroesophageal reflux after reconstruction of the esophagus with colon interposition. Wiad Lek 1997, 50, Suppl 1, 1: 322-325.

[51] Strutyńska-Karpińska M, Lewandowski A, Knast W, Markocka-Maczka K, Czapla L, Błaszczuk J. Comparative evaluation of postoperative complication in the reconstructive surgery of the esophagus. Wiad Lek 1999, 52:367-372.

[52] Milnerowicz S, Strutyńska-Karpińska M, Grabowski K, Lewandowski A. Long term results after esophagoplasty with the large and small bowel. Surg Childh Intern 1999, 3: 193-197.

[53] Neville WE, Najem AZ. Colon replacement of the esophagus for congenital and benign disease. Ann Thorac Surg 1983, 36: 626-633.

[54] Kovalenko PP, Chepurnoi GI. Comparative appraisal of esophagoplasty methods (clinical and experimental study). Chir 1978, 11: 51-57.

[55] Bernat M. Method of pharyngo-intestinal anastomosis in reconstruction of total retrosternal esophagus. Pol Przegl Chir 1979, 51: 673-678.

[56] Strutyńska-Karpińska M. Frequency of cervical anastomotic leaks after various types of oesophagoplasty – a retrospective study. Adv Clin Exp Med 2002, 11: 473-479.

[57] Strutyńska-Karpińska M, Ciesielska A, Błaszczuk J, Wierzbicki J, Zielony A, Taboła R. Evaluation of types of cervical anastomoses in oesophageal reconstructive surgery. Adv Clin Exp Med 2002, 11: 445-450.

[58] Stefan H. Esophageal replacement using the large intestine in children. Rozh Chir 1992, 71: 530-535.

[59] Bernat M. Effect of disorders of gastric emptying on the function of artificial esophagus made of the intestine. Pol Przegl Chir 1979, 51: 599-605.

[60] Clark J, Moraldi A, Moosa AR, Hall AW, DeMeester TR, Skinner DB. Functional evaluation of the interposed colon as an esophageal substitute. Ann Surg 1976, 183: 93-100.

[61] Orringer MB, Kirsh MM, Sloan H. New trends in esophageal replacement for benign disease. Ann Thorac Surg 1977, 23: 409-416.

[62] Miller H, Lam KH, Ong GB. Observations of pressure waves in stomach, jejunal, and colonic loops used to replace the oesophagus. Surgery 1975, 5: 543-551.

[63] Jezioro Z, Bernat M, Piegza S, Zimmer Z. Hemorrhagic, peptic esophagitis of an esophagus made from the colon. Pol Przegl Chir. 1967, 39: 1-6.

[64] Jezioro Z. Functional results and delayed complications following retrosternal surgery producing and esophagus from large intestine by my own method, 1950-1970. Pol Przegl Chir1977, 49: 1199-1205.

[65] Moreno-Oset E, Tomas-Ridocci M, Paris F,Mora F, Garcia-Zarza A, Molina R, Pastor J, Benages A. Motor activity of esophageal substitute (stomach, jejunal, and colon segments). Ann Thorac Surg 1986, 41: 515-519.

[66] Calleja IJ, Moreno E, Santoyo J, Gomez M, Navalon J, Arias J, Castellanos G, Solis JA. Long esophagoplasty: functional study. Hepatogastroenterol 1988, 35: 279-284.

[67] McLarty AJ, Deschamps C, Trastek VF, Allen MS, Pairolero PC, Harmsen WS. Esophageal resection for cancer of the esophagus: long-term function and quality of life. Ann Thorac Surg 1997, 63:1568-1572.

[68] Cherki S, Mabrut JY, Adham M, De La Roche E, Ducerf C, Gouillat C, Berard P, Baulieux J. Reinterventions for complication and defect of coloesophagoplasty. Ann Chir 2005, 130: 242-248.

[69] Dreuw B, Fass J, Titkowa S, Anurov M, Polivoda M, Ottinger AP, Schumpelick V. Colon interposition for esophageal replacement: isoperistaltic or antiperistaltic? Experimental results. Ann Thorac Surg 2001, 71:303-308.

[70] Mansour KA, Bryan FC, Carlson GW. Bowel interposition for esophageal replacement: twenty-five-year experience. Ann Thorac Surg 1997, 64: 752-756.

[71] Reffensperger JG, Luck SR, Reynolds M, Schwartz D. Intestinal bypass of the esophagus. J Pediatr Surg 1996, 31: 38-46.

[72] Popovici Z. A new philosophy in esophageal reconstruction with colon. Thirty-years experience. Dis Esophagus 2003, 16: 323-327.

[73] Pasalega M, Mesină C, Calotă F, Vălcea D, Nemes R, Burdescu C, Curcă T, Paraliov T, Mirea C, Tenea C, Vasile I. Coloesophagoplasty, a choice operation for postcaustic esophageal stenosis. Chirurgia (Bucur) 2004, 99: 515-521.

[74] Wormuth JK, Heitmiller RF. Esophageal conduit necrosis. Thorac Surg Clin 2006, 16: 11-22.

[75] Chirica M, Veyrie N, Munoz-Bongrand N, Zohar S, Halimi B, Celerier M, Cattan P, Sarfati E. Late morbidity after colon interposition for corrosive esophageal injury: risk factors, management, and outcome. A 20-years experience. Ann Surg 2010, 252:271-280.

Chapter 2

Esophageal Reconstruction with Small Intestine

1. Vascular anatomy of the small intestine

The small intestine as a whole, i.e. the jejunum and the ileum, is supplied with arterial blood by intestinal arteries (aa. jejunales and aa. ilei), which are branches of the superior mesenteric artery (a. mesenterica superior) and run together in the intestinal mesentery. Individual intestinal arteries, from 10 to 15 in number, referred to as main trunks, anastomose with each other by means of so-called vascular arcades. The outflow of venous blood belongs to the confluence of the portal vein and takes place in homonymous veins.

Numerous anatomical studies on vascular structure of the jejunum have demonstrated that only 30% of population reveals so-called adequate vascular system for esophageal reconstructions, which enables reconstructive surgery with a pedicled segment of the jejunum. Further 30% of population has definitely disadvantageous vascular anatomy in the aspect of reconstructive surgery, while the remaining individuals present with so-called intermediate arrangements, which only in few cases permit mobilization of a pedicled esophageal graft from this intestinal segment. Thus the use of the jejunum to create an esophageal graft is strictly conditioned by the possibility of mobilization of a long enough and well vascularized intestinal segment reaching up to the neck. The above mentioned individually differentiated vasculature of the mesojejunum is thus the key point allowing or excluding use of the jejunum for esophageal reconstruction.

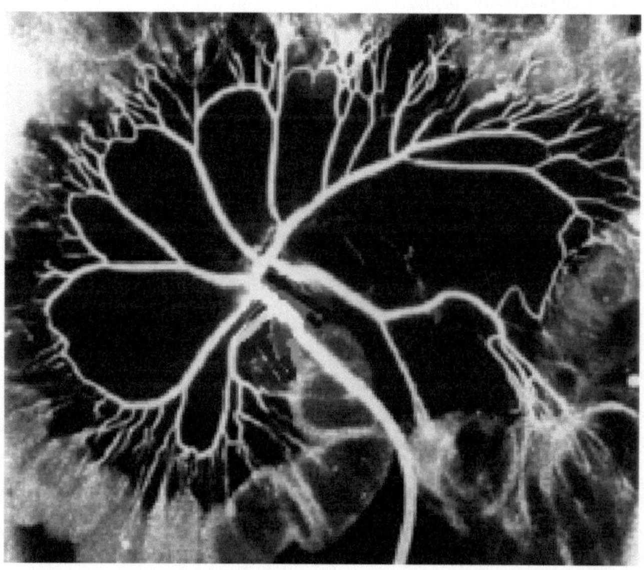

Figure 1 Angiogram of an adequate arterial system of the mesojejunum (well developed main vascular trunks connected by long and well developed arcades)

From the point of view of reconstructive surgery, the above-mentioned vasculature systems of the mesojejunum may be presented in the following way.

An adequate vasculature contains well developed, long vascular trunks, which anastomose between themselves by means of equally well developed and long arcades (Fig. 1).

An inadequate vascular system is such, in which the main vascular trunks either do not form anastomosing arcades, or between some of the trunks there are poorly developed arcades alternating with trunks with bushy architecture. Such systems may be observed in anatomical preparations of the small intestine, or intraoperatively (Fig. 2, 3).

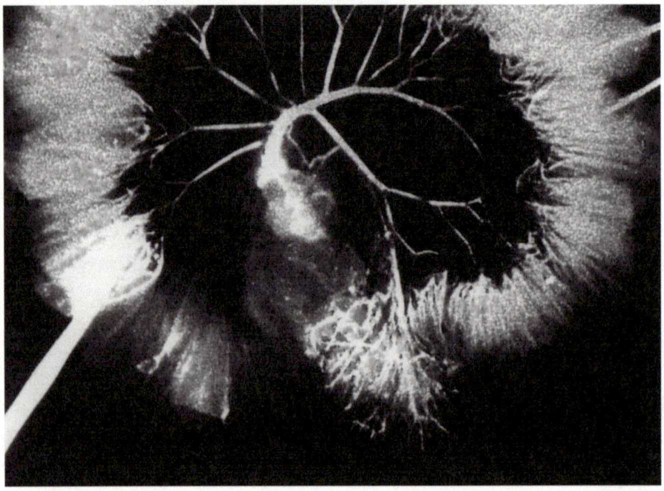

Figure 2 Angiogram of an inadequate arterial system of the mesojejunum (main vascular trunks do not form anastomosing arcades)

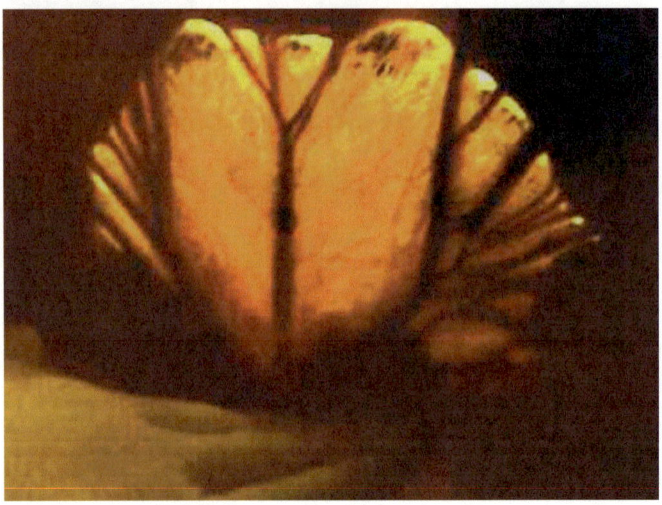

Figure 3 Intraoperative picture of an inadequate vasculature of the mesojejunum (main vascular trunks branch and do not form anastomosing arcades)

An intermediate system is a mixture of adequate and inadequate systems. With this type of vasculature, it is rarely possible to mobilize a long enough and well supplied segment of the jejunum on a vascular pedicle, even when the surgeon is equipped with highest quality skills. In such cases it is better to abandon this part of intestine and consider colon graft by means of one of the methods described in the chapter on esophageal reconstruction with colon.

2. Esophageal reconstructions using the jejunum

As presented in the previous chapter, reconstructive surgery using the jejunum consists of a number of consecutive stages: abdominal, cervical and thoracic.

The abdominal cavity is approached from upper midline incision reaching from the xiphoid process of the sternum to the umbilicus. Next first loops of the jejunum are exposed, starting from the duodenojejunal flexure, and the type of vasculature can be determined at this point. In order to enable visualization of the vasculature, the jejunum should be lifted upwards and its mesentery should be illuminated with a lateral source of light, so-called transillumination (Fig. 3). If vascular system appears adequate, the next step is to evaluate the efficacy of vascular anastomoses by means of a biological trial. Vascular forceps are clamped on the main vascular trunks which are to be cut below their bifurcation, starting from the 2nd intestinal artery in order to create conditions in which the selected and separated intestinal segment is supplied exclusively from this artery and vein which create the future vascular pedicle of the graft. Usually it is the 3rd or the 4th intestinal artery. If the vascular anastomoses in the selected intestinal segment are efficient, the intestine maintains natural colour and peristalsis. Disrupted blood supply is manifested by intense peristalsis and cyanosis or marble-like appearance of the intestine and lack of visible pulse in the distal straight vessels of the investigated intestinal segment. A precise evaluation of the adequacy of vasculature in the separated intestinal segment may be achieved by intraoperative ultrasound Doppler scanning.

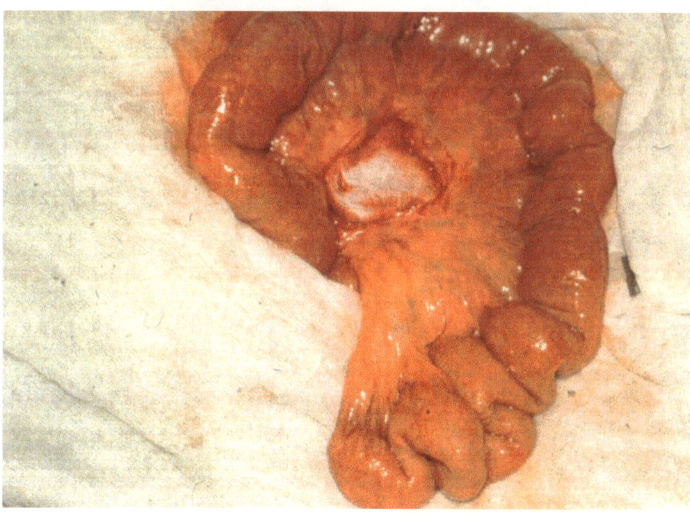

Figure 4 Intraoperative picture of onset of mobilization of a pedicled graft from the jejunum

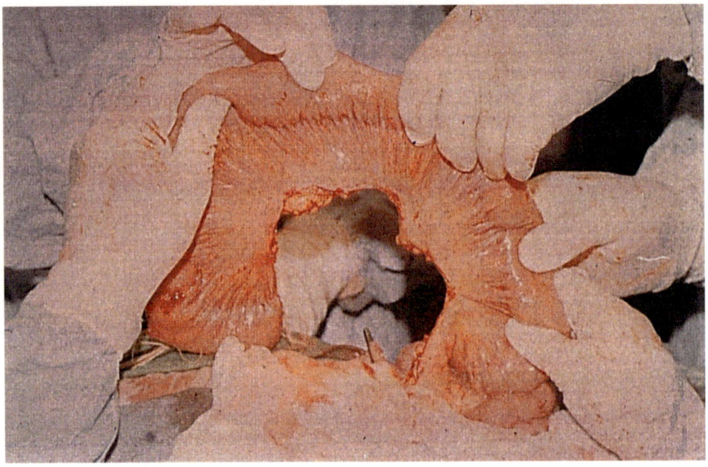

Figure 5 Intraoperative picture of continuation of mobilization of a pedicled graft from the jejunum

A positive biological trial means that the graft mobilization may be started. For this reason the vascular trunks, i.e. the second or the second and third intestinal artery and vein should be ligated and transected following prior clamping with forceps in the proximity to the site of their branching from the mesenteric vessels (Fig. 4, 5). It is important, as length of the vascular pedicle is crucial to obtain a long enough and well vascularized graft reaching up to the neck.

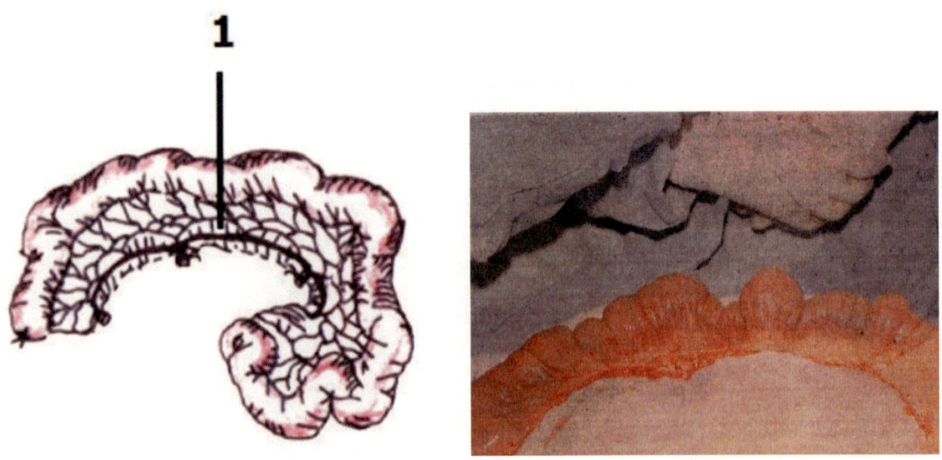

Figure 6 Diagram and intraoperative picture of a mobilized graft from the jejunum:
1 – vascular pedicle of the graft

Radial, Y-shaped incision of the mesenteric layer of the peritoneum with a 2-cm safety margin from the border vessels, i.e. arches anastomosing the transected trunks of the mobilized intestine allows to obtain a straight graft and at the same time it elongates its vascular pedicle. The next step involves full mobilization of the graft. The jejunum is transected 20 cm from the duodenojejunal flexure and in the caudal portion beyond the vascular trunk which forms the graft pedicle (Fig. 6). In order to obtain sufficient mobility of the created graft, a few-centimeter segment of the intestine is excised following parietal ligation and cutting of the terminal straight vessels in the caudal portion. This procedure is referred to as reduction in the distal portion of the graft (Fig. 7). The cephalic stump of the graft should be closed tight with a manual suture or stapled, and its caudal segment is closed with a temporary suture until it becomes anastomosed with the stomach. Thus created graft is covered with a surgical towel soaked in warm saline. Next continuity of the gastrointestinal tract within the abdominal cavity should be restored by anastomosing the jejunal stumps remaining after mobilization of the graft. During this procedure, the created graft should be observed periodically for blood supply.

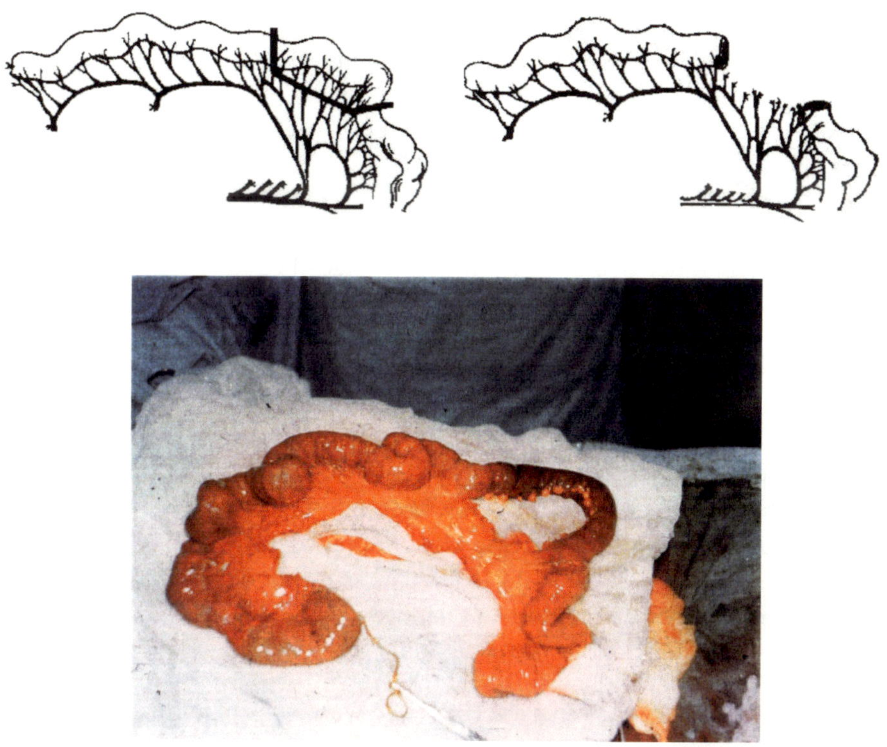

Figure 7 Diagram and intraoperative picture of full mobilization of the graft with prepared reduction of the intestine in caudal segment

The next activity at this stage of the surgery is to place the created graft in the epigastrium. There are several variants. The first of them, and most advantageous, is to move the graft beyond the colon and the stomach. This is the shortest route towards the neck and involves passing the mobilized graft together with its vascular pedicle through a slit in the transverse mesocolon and the lesser omentum from the mesogastrium to the epigastrium. Thanks to prior reduction of the intestine in the caudal portion, the graft is more mobile and the pedicle, which remains beyond the stomach, is well protected. However this variant cannot be applied in all the patients. This especially concerns individuals after extensive surgeries in the epigastrium. Then one of two possible variants of pull-through of the graft should be chosen. The first of them consists in passing the graft behind the colon and in front of the stomach. In comparison to the previous method, this modality is less advantageous and requires mobilization of a significantly longer intestinal segment. The main reason for this is the fact that the graft pedicle surrounds the greater curvature of the stomach and thus hampers mobility of the graft, what should be remembered at the beginning of graft mobilization. The last variant is the least advantageous. In this variant the graft is pulled in front of both, the colon and the stomach. It requires mobilization of even longer segment of the jejunum in comparison to the previous methods. Additionally, another drawback is that the vascular pedicle, which surrounds the transverse colon and the stomach, is exposed to pressure, what may disrupt blood circulation in the graft.

As can be understood from the surgical details presented above, every decision made at individual stages of the operation must be carefully balanced, as it affects the outcome of the reconstructive surgery.

After termination of the abdominal stage of mobilization and translocation of the graft to the epigastrium, the next activity is to construct a retrosternal canal and pull the graft through the canal to the neck. A detailed description of this stage of operation was presented in the previous chapter.

After placing the graft in the retrosternal canal, the next step is to anastomose its caudal portion with anterior wall of the prepyloric stomach. During this procedure a special attention should be paid to the blood supply to the portion of the graft which is exposed onto the neck. Normally supplied graft in the portion exposed onto the neck maintains peristalsis, reveals pulsation in the terminal intestinal vessels close to the intestinal wall, and the intestinal wall is shiny and pink. In cases any disturbances in blood supply to the portion exposed on the neck are noticed, the graft should be evacuated from the canal and the cause of obstructed blood flow should be immediately determined and removed.

In this place it is worth reminding that creation of the retrosternal canal, and especially translocation of the graft through the canal are associated with a risk of intestinal torsion around the vascular pedicle, suspension of the pedicle on the diaphragm at the site of the opening of the canal from the abdominal side, and in ultimate case, disruption of the graft's vascular pedicle. Disruption of the vascular pedicle is a severe complication, which is most commonly irreversible, and it thwarts the whole reconstructive surgery. In this case a trial to anastomose ruptured vessels may be undertaken, however a positive outcome is doubtful. In case of intestinal torsion around the pedicle, the twisting should be resolved, the intestine should be covered with a surgical towel soaked in warm saline, and after restoration of normal blood supply, the graft should be again pulled through the retrosternal canal. If the blood supply was disrupted through pressure of the diaphragm at the level of the inferior opening of the retrosternal canal, the diaphragm should be incised sagittally in the canal axis. In this way the canal opening is widened and the pressure on the graft pedicle - relieved.

When the graft is anastomosed with the stomach, and blood supply to the cervical portion of the graft remains normal, the final stage of the reconstructive surgery, i.e. esophageal-intestinal anastomosis on the neck may start. Cervical anastomosis is the last, but at the same time extremely important stage of the reconstructive surgery, as it exerts a significant effect on the future function of the substitutive esophagus. Erroneously performed cervical anastomosis may be the reason of disturbances on swallowing, and in ultimate cases, of occlusion of the substitutive esophagus. The most advantageous is the end-side to side anastomosis of the cervical esophagus with the lateral intestinal wall. It is broad enough and it has a beneficial effect on the future function of the substitutive esophagus. In order to prevent the cephalic portion of the graft from forming an inclining downwards diverticulum, 1-2 sutures should be placed to suspend the stump of the cervical part of the graft on the sternocleidomastoid muscle (Fig. 8).

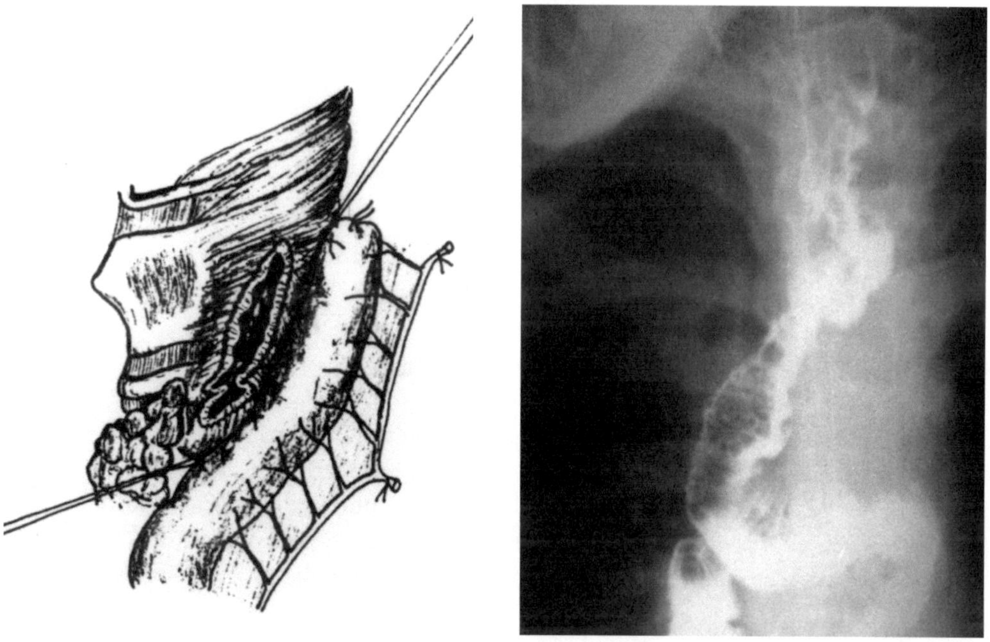

Figure 8 Diagram and radiogram (lateral projection) of cervical end-side to side anastomosis (the sutures run diagonally from behind and up towards the front and below)

After this stage, suturing the abdominal and cervical layers terminates the reconstructive surgery.

Recapitulating the above described esophageal reconstruction with the jejunum, it should be stressed that it has several advantages. The substitutive esophagus resumes excellent function, what is associated with the properties of the jejunum. Peristalsis is vivid, what favours quick and efficient passage of the content through the substitutive esophagus and prevents reflux. Moreover, translocation of the graft through the retrosternal canal and anastomosis with the cervical esophagus is easier in comparison to the colon. Finally, the intestinal defect in the abdominal cavity is minimal.

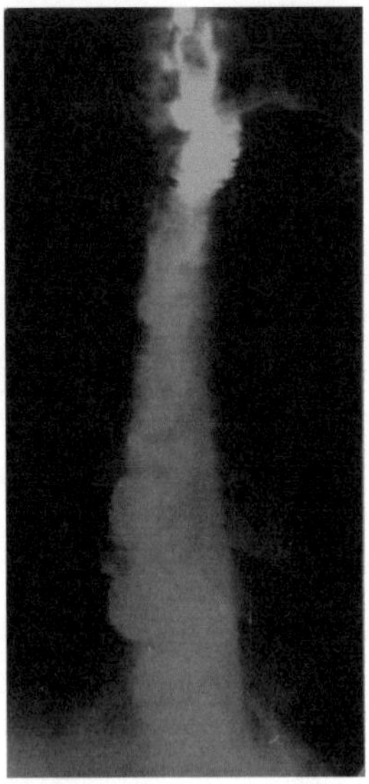

Figure 9 Radiogram of a substitutive esophagus created from the jejunum (A-P projection)

Follow up examinations immediately after the surgery as well as remote observations confirm an excellent function of thus performed esophageal reconstruction (Fig. 9).

3. Esophageal reconstructions using the ileum

Discussing reconstructive surgery with the use of the small intestine, it should be stressed that not only the jejunum may be used for esophageal reconstruction. The knowledge of modalities presented below may be useful in cases in which, due to anatomical conditions, reconstructive surgery using another portion of the intestine may appear unfeasible. Thus it seems reasonable to recollect anatomical details of vascularization in the ileocaecal angle.

The ileocaecal vessels, which run in the mesenteric root of the small intestine downwards and to the right, are responsible for blood supply to the terminal portion of the ileum, the caecum, and the vermiform appendix. Through the iliac branches they join with terminal arteries and veins of the intestine departing from the superior mesenteric vessels, and through the colon branch with arteries and veins of the right colon (Fig. 10).

Adequate vascular system within the terminal portion of the ileum and the right colon may be used to mobilize an isoperistaltic graft by means of three modalities:

1. from the ileum on ileocolic vascular pedicle;
2. from the ileum and caecum on ileocolic vascular pedicle;
3. from the terminal portion of the ileum, the caecum, and part of the ascending colon on right or middle colic vascular pedicle.

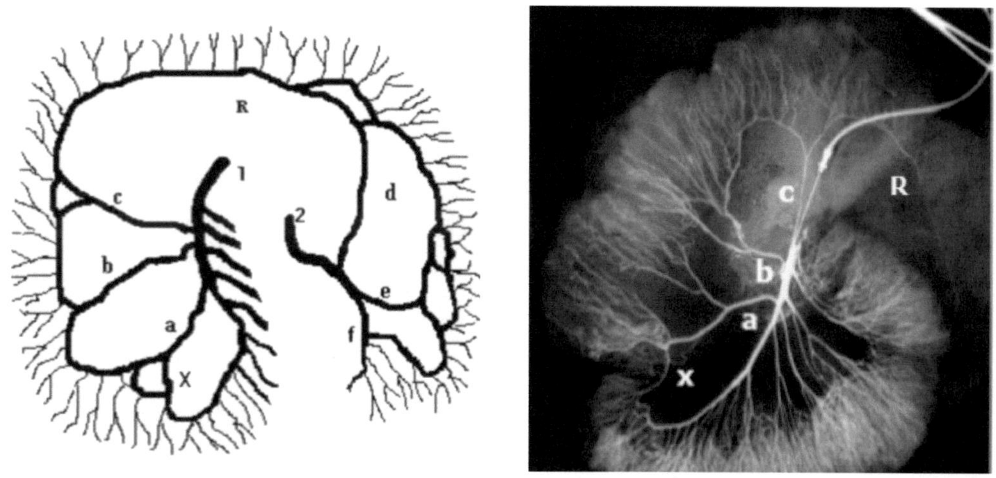

Figure 10 Diagram and angiogram of vasculature in the terminal portion of the ileum and the right colon. Diagram: 1 – art. mesenterica superior, a – art. ileocolica, b – art. colica dextra, c – art. colica media, X – ramus ilicus art. Ileocolicae, R – arcus Riolani. Angiogram: ball needle inserted to art. mesenterica superior, a – art. ileocolica, b – art. colica dextra, c – art. colica media, X – ramus ilicus art. Ileocolicae, R – arcus Riolani

Choice of one of the above modalities is closely associated and conditioned by an adequate and fully efficacious vasculature, which is able to provide the best possible blood supply to the future graft.

3.1. Esophageal reconstruction with the use of the ileum alone

The ileum is extremely rarely used in esophageal reconstructions due to a short mesoileum and running in several rows, short arcades anastomosing intestinal vessels. Thus adequate evaluation of the vascular efficacy in this portion of the intestine is very difficult even for an experienced surgeon. Another reason is associated with the fact that a graft made from the ileum in general has a tortuous course, i.e. there is a significant excess of the ileum in relation to the mesentery, what exerts a negative effect on the function of the substitutive esophagus, despite peristalsis characteristic for the small intestine. Thus it should be emphasized decidedly that this type of reconstructive surgery should be considered only in cases in which, due to anatomical conditions, reconstruction with another segment of the intestine is impossible. However awareness of this surgical modality is a chance for patients to regain the possibility of oral alimentation.

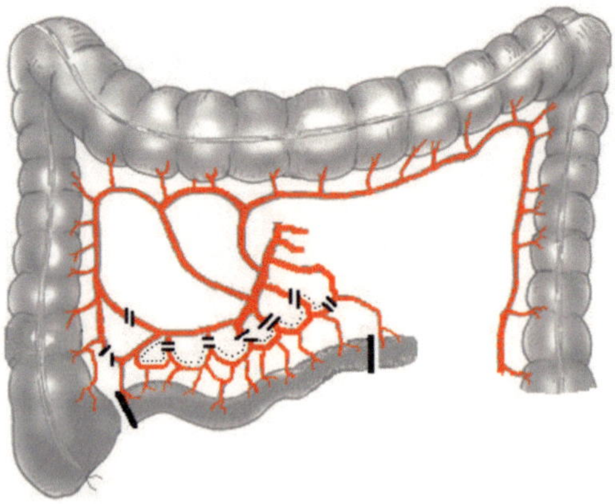

Figure 11 Diagram of mobilization of the ileum graft on ileocolic vascular pedicle

The surgical technique is as follows. The abdominal cavity is approached from the upper midline incision passing by the umbilicus on the right side and going several centimeters below. Next the caecum, the ascending colon together with the ileocolic vessels, and the terminal portion of the ileum together with its mesentery and terminal branches of the superior mesenteric vessels should be prepared and separated from the posterior abdominal wall. Thus mobilized portion of the intestine enables a detailed evaluation of the vasculature in the mobilized intestinal segment. In case circulation is found adequate, i.e. ileocolic vessels are long, well developed and form wide and firm arcades anastomosing with the right colic vessels and, through the iliac branch, with vessels in the terminal portion of the ileum, a biological trial should be undertaken. The trunks of the terminal portion of the ileum which is to be transected, as well as the colic branch of the ileocolic vessels are clamped with vascular forceps just at its departure from the main ileocolic trunk. The selected terminal segment of the ileum is thus supplied only from the ileocolic vessels.

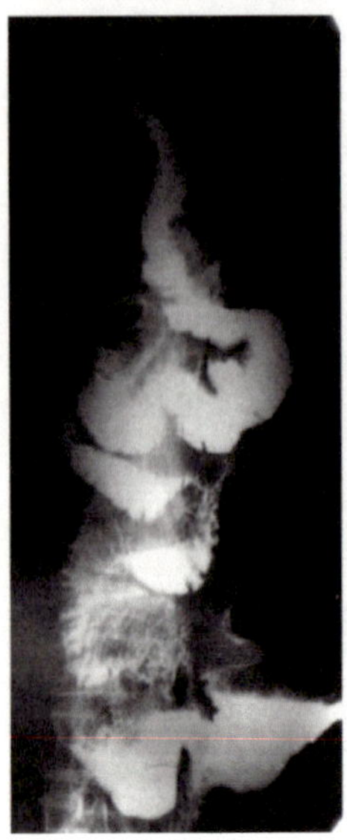

Figure 12 Radiogram of a substitutive esophagus created from the ileum (A-P projection)

A positive result of the biological trial allows continuation of the operation. However it should be remembered that length of the vascular pedicle is crucial for obtaining a long enough graft. As the mesoileum is short, and the main vascular trunks form several rows of arcades, mobilization of the ileum is much more difficult in comparison to the jejunum; moreover, it requires mobilization of a relatively long intestinal segment, which would reach the neck without tension. Mobilization of the graft starts from ligation and transection of the vessels which were previously clamped, with a special attention paid not to damage the continuity of the parietally placed arcades between ileocolic vessels and vessels of the terminal portion of the ileum. The graft is fully mobilized when the ileum is transected in the caecal portion and in the proximal segment at a level which is considered sufficient to obtain a required length of the graft (Fig. 11). Thus the graft, created totally from the ileum, has an ileocolic vascular pedicle and, after being pulled through the retrosternal canal, will be in isoperistaltic position. When the graft mobilization is completed, the vermiform appendix is resected. Further stages of the surgery, as described previously, involve formation of a retrosternal canal in which the graft is placed, reconstruction of the gastrointestinal continuity in the abdomen, i.e. anastomosing the ileum remaining after mobilization of the graft with the caecum and anastomosing the graft with the stomach and the cervical esophagus. The presented surgical modality was proposed by Bernat in 1988, and the patients operated on with this technique regained the possibility of nutrition through the mouth. (Fig. 12).

3.2. Esophageal reconstruction using the ileum and the caecum

The below presented technique for esophageal reconstruction is an original modality developed and proposed by Jezioro in 1958. It is based on an adequate vascular system for esophageal reconstruction in the region of the ileocolic angle. The main advantage of this surgical technique involves the use of a shorter segment of the ileum in comparison to the modality described above. Moreover, the caecum together with Bauhin's valve are included in the graft and create its caudal portion, at the same time performing the function of an antireflux mechanism.

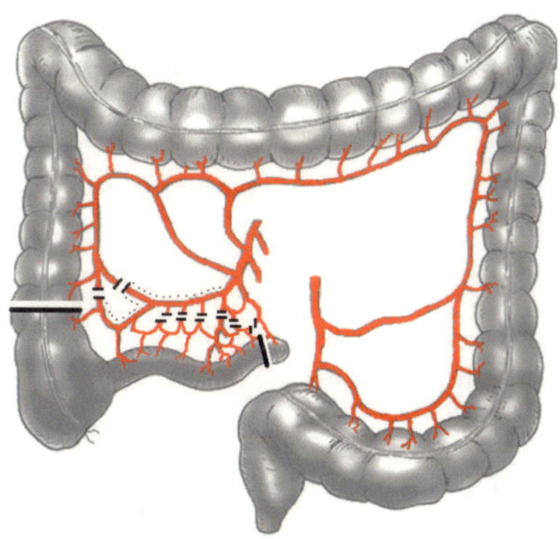

Figure 13 Diagram of mobilization of the graft from the ileum and the caecum on ileocolic vascular pedicle

The surgical technique is similar to the above-described modality of esophageal reconstruction with the ileum, the main difference lying in this that the colic branch of the iloecolic vessels should be ligated and transected just at the level of ramification of the right colic trunk in order to provide blood supply to the caecum. Thus an isoperistaltic graft is created on an ileocolic vascular pedicle. Mobilization of the ileum is similar to that described for the esophageal reconstruction with the ileum alone. But in this surgical modality the segment of the ileum is slightly shorter, and the caecum, as mentioned above, is included into the graft and creates its caudal portion (Fig. 13, 14). The vermiform appendix is resected after mobilization of the graft.

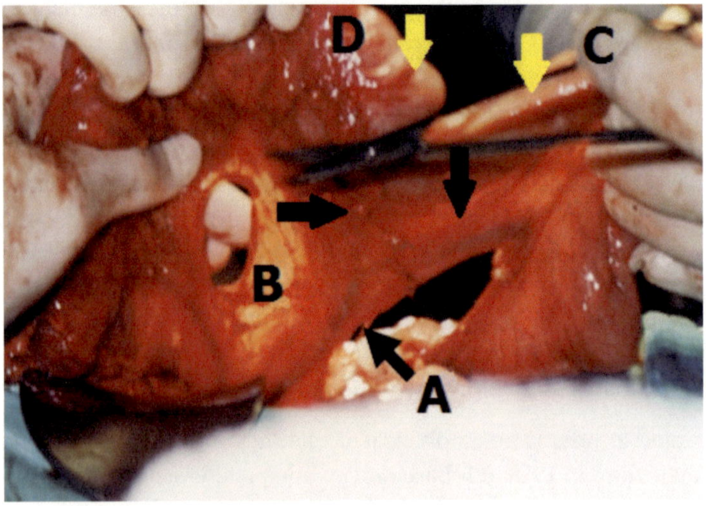

Figure 14 Intraoperative picture of mobilization of graft from the ileum and the caecum on ileocolic vascular pedicle: A – graft pedicle, B – ramus colicus art. ileocolecae, C – terminal segment of the ileum, D – the caecum

The mobilized intestinal segment is passed behind the colon and the stomach to the retrosternal canal. The ileum, forming the upper portion of the graft, is exposed to the neck and anastomosed with the cervical esophagus, and the caecum is anastomosed with the anterior wall of the prepyloric stomach. The intestinal passage in the abdominal cavity is reconstructed by anastomosis between the part of the ileum remaining after mobilization of the graft and the ascending colon. Anastomosis of the ileum exposed on the neck with the cervical esophagus completes the operation.

The presented technique of reconstructive surgery has a number of advantages. The cephalic portion of the graft is formed from the small intestine with a vivid peristalsis. On the other hand, the caecum together with the ileocolic valve, as mentioned before, plays the function of an antireflux barrier.

The drawbacks include relative tortuosity of the graft, what elongates the passage through the esophageal substitute.

Clinical follow up at a remote time indicated that the function of so created esophagus may be considered good (Fig. 15).

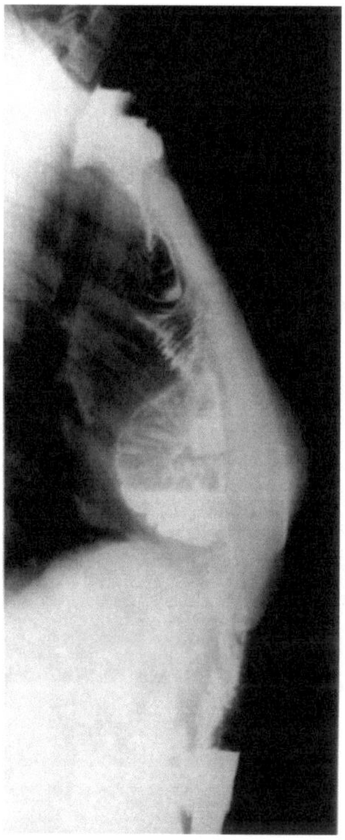

Figure 15 Radiogram of substitutive esophagus from the ileum and the caecum (lateral projection)

3.3. Esophageal reconstruction using the ileum, the caecum and part of the ascending colon

The last of the surgical modalities with the use of the ileum involves mobilization of a graft consisting of the ileum in its cephalic portion and from the caecum and part of the ascending colon in the caudal portion. The described below technique differs from the two techniques presented previously in this that the distal portion of the graft is made from the caecum and a short segment of the ascending colon, while the pedicle includes the right or middle colic vessels.

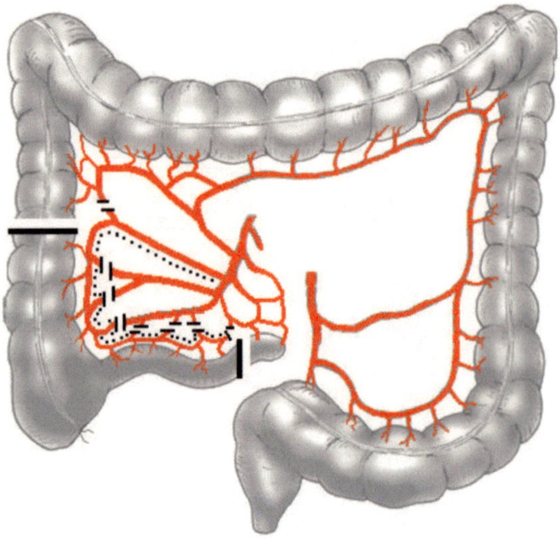

Figure 16 Diagram of mobilization of graft from the ileum, the caecum and part of the ascending colon on middle colic vascular pedicle

This variant of reconstructive surgery is possible in patients with effective vasculature systems between vessels in the terminal portion of the ileum and the right colon. Then an isoperistaltic graft may be created on a pedicle of right or middle colic vessels. However it should be remembered that a graft on right colic vascular pedicle has a shorter pedicle than a graft pedicled on middle colic vessels.

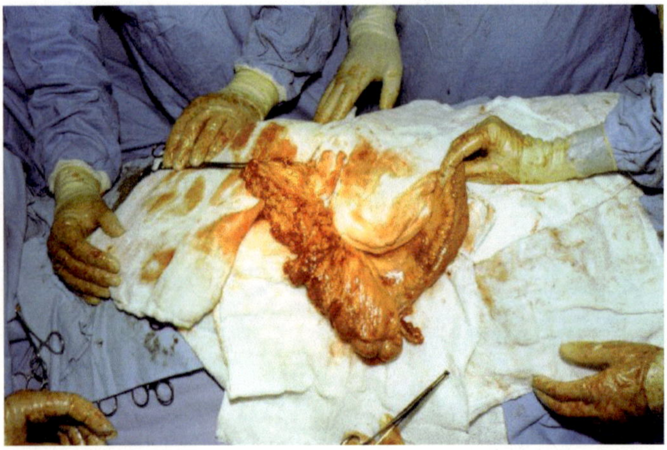

Figure 17 Intraoperative picture of mobilization of terminal portion of the ileum and the right colon

The surgical technique differs slightly from the two previously described surgical modalities. After laparotomy, the terminal portion of the ileum and the right colon must be mobilized. If the adequacy of vasculature in the terminal ileum and the right colon is ascertained macroscopically, and a biological trial of the graft pedicle on the right colic vessels is also positive, the ileocolic vessels and the trunks of the vessels in the terminal ileum are ligated and transected with anastomosing arcades left intact. The ascending colon is transected beyond ramification of the right colic vessels, and the ileum – at a distance of 20 cm from the caecum. In cases in which a longer graft is necessary, also the right colic vessels should be ligated and transected, and the graft should be pedicled on middle colic vessels. In this variant the mobilized segment of the ileum is shorter than in the two previously described esophageal reconstructions with the use of the ileum, or the ileum and the caecum, and it is straight (Fig. 16, 17, 18). The vermiform appendix is resected in a routine manner following full mobilization of the graft.

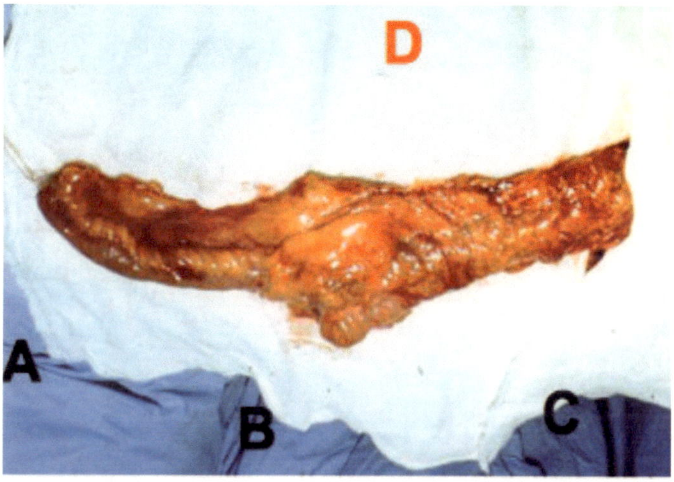

Figure 18 Intraoperative picture of graft from the ileum, the caecum and part of the ascending colon on middle colic vascular pedicle: A – terminal portion of the ileum, B – the caecum, C – the ascending colon, D – vascular pedicle

The remaining surgical procedures are the same as presented in previous chapters. The mobilized graft is pulled behind the colon and the stomach to the retrosternal canal. The remaining stump of the ileum is connected to the residual right colon. The caudal portion of the graft, i.e. the ascending colon is anastomosed to the anterior wall of the prepyloric stomach, while the cephalic portion, which has been created from the terminal segment of the ileum - to the cervical esophagus.

The above presented modality of esophageal reconstruction has many advantages. The cephalic portion of the esophageal substitute is created from the small intestine with a vivid peristalsis, and Bauhin's valve, which is located in the middle of the graft, may be considered an antireflux barrier. Moreover, the abdominal defect remaining after mobilization of the graft is relatively slight.

The function of thus created esophageal substitute is effective, what finds confirmation on remote follow up (Fig. 19).

Recapitulating the above-presented modalities of esophageal reconstructions with the use of the small intestine, it should be underlined that they extend our knowledge on the possibilities of using the small intestine for esophageal reconstruction.

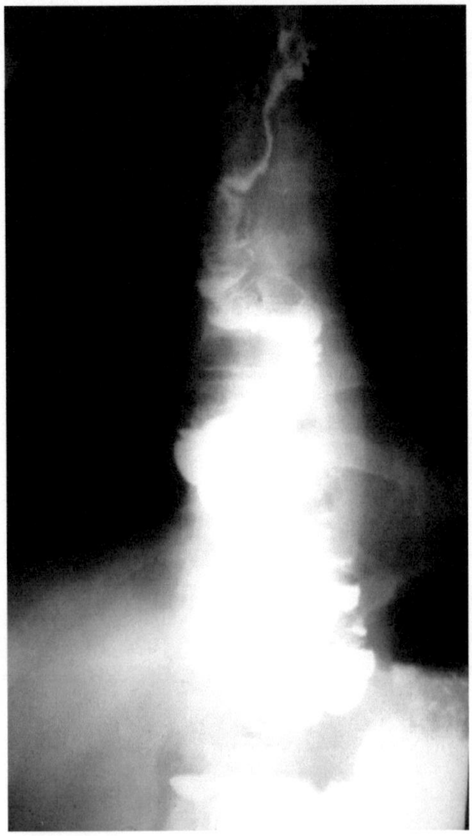

Figure 19 Radiogram of substitutive esophagus from the ileum, the caecum and part of the ascending colon (A-P projection)

4. References

[1] Roux C. L'oesophago-jejuno-gastrome, nouvelle operation pour retrecissement infranchissable de l'oesophage. La Semaine Medicale 1907, 27, 4, 37.

[2] Rydygier L. O plastyce przełyku z opisem preparatu anatomicznego po operacji Roux'a. Gazeta Lekarska 1909, rok XLIV, tom XXIX, ser.II,49,1089.

[3] Rienhoff WF Jr. Intrathoracic esophagojejunostomy for lesions of the upper third of the esophagus. South Med J 1946, 39: 928-940.

[4] Yudin SS. The surgical construction of 80 cases of artificial esophagus. Surg Gynec Obst 1944, 78: 561-.583.

[5] Harrison AW. Transthoracic Small Bowel Substitution in High Stricture of the Esophagus. J Thorac Surg 1949, 18: 316-326.

[6] Robertson R, Sarjeant TR. Reconstruction of the esophagus. J Thorac Surg 1950, 20: 689-705.

[7] Gasiński J. Esophageal surgery according to 121 cases. Pol Tyg Lek 1955, 10: 1269-1273.

[8] Dryjski J. Retrosternal intrapleural formation of artificial esophagus with jejunum in caustic stenosis caused by sodium hydroxide. Pol Tyg Lek 1957, 12: 1345-1357.

[9] Rauber-Kopsch F. Lehrbuch und Atlas der Anatomie des Menschen. Abteilung 3. Georg Thieme, Verlag, Leipzig 1923.

[10] Michels NA. Blood supply of the upper abdominal organs with a descriptive atlas. Philadelphia PA: Lippincott, 1955.

[11] Schumacher GH. Human topographic anatomy. Ed 1, Volumed, Wrocław, Poland, 1994, p 192-194.

[12] Bussemaker JB, Lindeman J. Comparison of methods to determine viability of small intestine. Ann Surg 1972, 176: 97-101.

[13] Zingerman LS, Khaliulin AI, Kudinov AA, Pogodina AN, Abakumov MM. Experience with using selective angiography of the mesenteric arteries in patients with cicatricial esophageal stenosis. Vestn Khir Im II Grek 1988, 140: 19-22.

[14] Horgan PG, Gorey TF. Operative assessment of intestinal viability. Surg Clin North Am 1992, 72: 143-155.

[15] Horton KM, Fishman EK. CT angiography of the mesenteric circulation. Radiolog Clin North AM 2010, 48: 331-345.

[16] Jezioro Z, Kuś H. Retrosternal esophagoplasty with jejunal graft in children. Zentralbl Chir 1957, 82: 425-436

[17] Jezioro Z, Kuś H. Retrosternal transplantation of the small intestine in formation of the esophagus. Pol Przegl Chir 1957, 29: 301-323.

[18] Wright CB, Hobson RW. Prediction of intestinal viability using Doppler ultrasound technics. Am J Surg 1975, 129: 642-645.

[19] Wright CB, Cuschieri A. Jejunal interposition for benign esophageal disease. Ann Surg 1987, 205: 54-60.

[20] Bernat M. Usefulness of the jejunum in fashioning whole retrosternal esophagus anastomosed with larynx. Pol Przegl Chir 1977, 49: 1147-1153.

[21] Bernat M. Method of pharyngo-intestinal anastomosis in reconstruction of total retrosternal esophagus. Pol Przegl Chir 1979, 51: 673-678.

[22] Belousov EV, Zadorozhny AA, Baidala PG, Tun VG, Bashirova LV. Coagulative alternations of blood circulation in transplant and their prophylacties in small intestine esophagoplasty. Vest Khir im II Grek 1987, 7: 120-123.

[23] Cusick EL, Batchelor AA, Spicer RD. Development of a technique for jejunal interposition in long-gap esophageal atresia. J Pediatr Surg 1993, 28: 990-994.

[24] Deschamps C. Use of colon and jejunum as possible esophageal replacements. Chest Surg Clin N Am 1995, 5: 555-569.

[25] Strutyńska-Karpińska M.: Operacje wytwórcze przełyku z jelita cienkiego. Biblioteka Pol Przegl Chir, tom 13, Warszawa 2000.

[26] Bax NM, van der Zee DC. Jejunal pedicle grafts for reconstruction of the esophagus in children. J Pediatr Surg 2007, 42: 363-369.

[27] Maish MS, DeMeester SR. Indications and technique of colon and jejunal interpositions for esophageal disease. Surg Clin North Am 2005, 85: 505-514.

[28] Randjelovic T, Dikic S, Filipovic B, Gacic D, Bilanovic D, Stanisavljevic N. Short-segment jejunoplasty: the option treatment in the management of benign esophageal stricture. Dis Esophagus 2007, 20: 239-246.

[29] Negre E, Coulon P. Presternal ileum and right colon for benign esophageal stenosis. Very long-term checking. J Chir (Paris) 1984, 121: 639-642.

[30] Celerier M, Tran Ba Huy P, Sarfati E, Gossot D. Esophagoplasty by right ileocolic graft technic. Treatment of caustic lesions of the hypopharynx. Chirurgie 1986, 112: 591-595.

[31] Strutyńska-Karpińska M. Studies on the vascularization of the ileum and the right half of the colon in view of the possibilities of employing the above intestinal segments in reconstructive operations of the entire esophagus. Pol Przegl Chir 1995, 67: 1204-1213.

[32] Touloukian RJ, Tellides G. Retrosternal ileocolic esophageal replacement in children revisited. Antireflux role of the ileocecal valve. J Thorac Cardiovasc Surg 1994, 107: 1067-1072.

[33] Bothereau H, Munoz-Bongrand N, Lambert B, Montemagno S, Cattan P, Sarfati E. Esophageal reconstruction after caustic injury: is there still a place for right coloplasty? Am J Surg 2007, 193: 660-664.

[34] Kerlin P, Zinmeister A, Phillips S. Motor responses to food of the ileum, proximal colon, and distal colon of healthy humans. Gastroenterolog. 1983, 84: 762-770.

[35] Del Poli M, Mioli P, Gasparri G, Csalegno PA, Camandona M, Bronda M, Albertino B, Cassolino P. Functional study of intestinal trasnsplants after esophagectomy. Minerva Chir 1991, 46: 241-245.

[36] Miller H, Lam KH, Ong GB. Observations of presure waves in stomach, jejunal, and colonic loops used to replace the esophagus. Surgery 1975, 78: 543-551.

[37] Moreno-Osset E, Tomas-Ridocci M, Paris F, Mora F, Garcia-Zarza A, Molina R, Pastor J, Benager A. Motor activity of esophageal substitute (stomach, jejunal, and colon segments). Ann Thorac Surg 1986, 41: 515-519.

[38] Doki Y, Okada K, Miyata H, Yamasaki M, Fujiwara Y, Takiguchi S, Yasuda T, Hirao T, Nagano H, Monden M. Long-term and short-term evaluation of esophageal reconstruction using the

colon or the jejunum in esophageal cancer patients after gastrectomy. Dis Esophagus 2008, 21: 132-138.

[39] Buntain WL, Payne WS Lynn HB. Esophageal reconstruction for benign dissease: a long term appraisal. Am Surg 1980, 46: 67-79.

[40] Carlson GW, Anderson TM, Galloway JR, Monsour KA. Salvage of colon interposition by antethoracic free jejunal transfer. Ann Thorac Surg 1994, 58: 1523-1525.

[41] Chien KY, Wang PY, Lu KS. Esophagoplasty for corrosive stricture of the esophagus: an analysis of 60 cases. Ann Surg 1974, 197: 510-515.

[42] Chróścicki S, Towpik E. Esophageal stenosis after chemical burn – surgical treatment and discussion of our cases. Pol Przegl Chir 1980, 52: 681-687.

[43] Clarc J, Moraldi F, Moosa AR, Hall AW, DeMeester TR, Skinner DB. Functional evaluation of interposed colon as an esophageal substitute. Ann Surg 1976, 183: 93-100.

[44] Gerzic ZB, Knezevic JB, Milicevic MN, Jovanowic BK. Esophagocoloplasty in the management of postcorrosive strictures of the esophagus. Ann Surg 1990, 211: 329-336.

[45] Gossot D, Lefebvre JF. Ischaemic atrophy of the cervical portion of a substernal transplant: successful reconstruction using a syntetic restorable tube. Br J Surg 1988, 75: 801- 802.

[46] Grabowski K, Lewandowski A, Moroń K, Strutyńska-Karpińska M, Błaszczuk J, Machała R. Pleural hernia of an esophageal graft late postoperative complication. Wiad Lek. 1997, 50 Suppl 1, 1:339-343.

[47] Hirabayashi S, Miyata M, Shoji M, Shibusawa H. Reconstruction of the thoracic esophagus, with extended jejunum used as a substitute, with the aid of microvascular anastomosis. Surgery 1993, 113: 515-519.

[48] Jacob L, Rabary O, Boudaoud S, Payen D, Sarfaty E, Gossot D, Rolland E, Eurin B, Celerier M. Usefulness of perioperative pulsed Doppler flowmetry in predicting postoperative local ischaemic complications after ileocolic esophagoplasty. J Thorac Cardiovasc Surg 1992, 104: 385-390.

[49] Jezioro Z.: Wytworzenie przełyku z jelita krętego i kątnicy. Monografia. PZWL Warszawa 1960.

[50] Kurstin RD, Soltanzedeh H, Hobson RW, Wright CB. Ultrasonic blood flow assessment in coloesophageal bypass procedures. Arch.Surg. 1977, 112: 270-272.

[51] Kuś H. On a radilogical method in the study of mesenteric vessels in anatomical preparations. Pol Przegl Chir 1961, 25: 451-458.

[52] Kuś H. Experimental transplantation of isolated intestinal segments. Zentralbl Chir 1961, 86:1236-1242.

[53] Omura K, Misaki T, Urayama H, Ishida F, Watanabe Y. Composite reconstruction of the esophagus. J Surg Oncol 1993, 52: 18-20.

[54] Schumpelic V, Drew B, Ophoff K, Fass J. Esophageal replacement - indications, technique, results. Leber Magen Darm. 1995, 25: 21-26.

[55] Shiraha S, Matsumoto H, Terada M, Noguchi J, Sankoyji T, Hayaschi M. Motility studies of the cervical esophagus with intrathoracic gastric conduit after esophagectomy. Scand J Thorac Cardiovasc Surg 1992, 26: 119123.

[56] Strutyńska-Karpińska M. Causes of blood perfusion disturbances in pedunculated intestinal grafts employed in reconstructive procedures of the esophagus. Pol Przegl Chir 1993, 65: 1185-1190.

[57] Strutyńska-Karpińska M.: Sposób wytworzenia całego zamostkowego przełyku z jelita krętego, ślepego i części wstępnicy na szypule naczyń okrężniczych prawych lub środkowych. Praca habilitacyjna. Akad. Med. Wrocław 1995.

[58] Strutyńska-Karpińska M. Retrosternal canal in reconstructive procedures of the entire esophagus. Pol Przegl Chir 1997, 69: 1191-1196.

[59] Strutyńska-Karpińska M. Early postoperative complications in reconstructive operations of the esophagus. Pol Przegl Chir 1997, 69: 677-685.

[60] Horton KM, Fishman EK. CT angiography of the mesenteric circulation. Radiol Clin North Am 2010, 48:331-345.

[61] Zadorozhny AA, Baidala PG. Reconstructive operations on the artificial esophagus. Vestn Khir Im II Grek 1993, 151: 78-81.

[62] Yamamoto Y, Nohira K, Shintomi Y, Yoshida T, Minakawa H, Okushiba S, Fukuda S, Inuyama Y, Hosokawa M. Mesenteric flap in free jejunal transfers: a versatile technique for head and neck reconstruction. Head Neck 1995, 17: 213-218.

[63] Omura K, Urayama H, Kanehira E, Kaito K, Ohta K, Ishida Y, Takizawa M, Sumitomo H, Watanabe Y. Reconstruction of the thoracic esophagus using jejunal pedicle with vascular anastomoses. J Surg Oncol 2000, 75: 217-219.

[64] Maish MS, DeMeester SR. Indications and technique of colon and jejunal interpositions for esophageal disease. Surg Clin North Am 2005, 85: 505-514.

[65] Takushima A, Momosawa A, Asato H, Aiba E, Harii K. Double vascular pedicled free jejunum transfer for total esophageal reconstruction. J Reconstr Microsurg 2005, 21: 5-10.

[66] Bax NM, van der Zee DC. Jejunal pedicle grafts for reconstruction of the esophagus in children. J Pediatr Surg 2007, 42: 363-369.

[67] Numajiri T, Fujiwara T, Nishino K, Sowa Y, Uenaka M, Masuda S, Fujiwara H, Nakai S, Hisa Y. Double vascular anastomosis for safer free jejunal transfer in unfavorable conditions. J Reconstr Microsurg 2008, 24: 531-536.

[68] Doki Y, Okada K, Miyata H, Yamasaki M, Fujiwara Y, Takiguchi S, Yasuda T, Hirao T, Nagano H, Monden M. Long-term and short-term evaluation of esophageal reconstruction using the colon or the jejunum in esophageal cancer patients after gastrectomy. Dis Esophagus 2008, 21: 132-138.

[69] Poh M, Selber JC, Skoracki R, Walsh GL, Yu P.Technical challenges of total esophageal reconstruction using a supercharged jejunal flap. Ann Surg 2011, 253: 1122-1129.

[70] Yasuda T, Shiozaki H. Esophageal reconstruction using a pedicled jejunum with microvascular augmentation. Ann Thorac Cardiovasc Surg 2011, 17: 103-109.

[71] Matsumoto H, Hirai T, Kubota H, Murakami H, Higashida M, Hirabayashi Y. Safe esophageal reconstruction by ileocolic interposition. Dis Esophagus 2012, 25: 195-200 (2011, Epub ahead of print doi:10.1111/j.1442-2050.2011.01232.x.).

Modifications and Complex Esophageal Reconstructions

1. Modifications of esophageal reconstructions

Esophageal reconstructions with the use of pedicled intestinal segments are difficult procedures and require perfect mastering of the surgical technique. However, despite excellent professional skills of the surgeon, in view of individually differentiated and not always adequate vasculature in the region of the small and large intestine, there may always occur intraoperative difficulties in obtaining long enough and at the same time well supplied with blood graft.

For this reason it is seems reasonable to present various management modalities providing a positive outcome to the reconstructive surgery. Since reconstructions with the use of free intestinal flaps and vascular anastomosis are not the subject of the report, they will not be discussed here.

Below are presented following modifications and complex reconstrucive surgeries:

- Single and double resection of redundant intestine
- Double-pedicle esophageal reconstructions
- Secondary mobilization of a pedicled intestinal graft

1.1. Resection of redundant intestine

The resection of redundant intestine is performed for two reasons. The first includes increasing mobility of the graft, the second reason is to improve blood supply to the mobilized intestinal segment.

A. Single resection of redundant intestine

This type of resection, so-called single resection, concerns the caudal portion of the mobilized graft. The surgical technique is relatively simple and involves parietal ligature and transection of straight vessels followed by resection of a 2-3 cm segment of the intestine in the caudal portion of the graft. Continuity of the graft pedicle remains intact (Fig. 1, 2).

The above-presented modification provides a double advantage. Resection of few-centimeter long intestinal segment in the caudal portion of the graft increases mobility of the mobilized intestinal segment. At the same time, resection of a few-centimeter intestinal segment in the peripheral portion of the graft, with unchanged source of blood supply, improves blood supply to the mobilized intestinal segment.

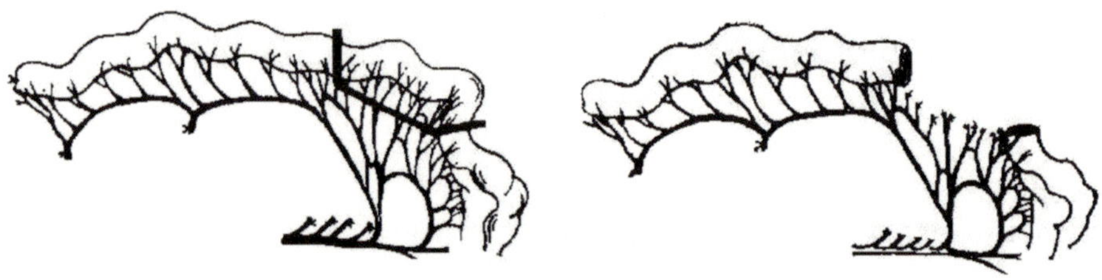

Figure 1 Diagram of single resection of redundant intestine in the caudal portion of the graft

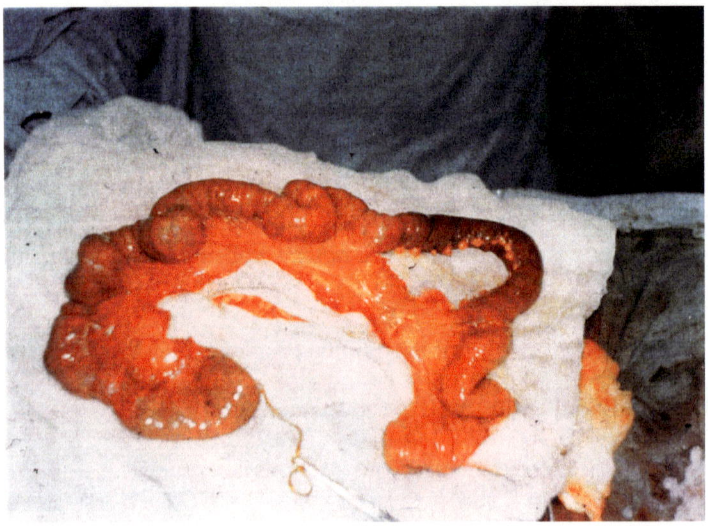

Figure 2 Intraoperative picture of prepration to single resection of redundant intestine in the caudal portion of the graft

B. Double resection of redundant intestine

Double resection of redundant intestine involves resection of redundant intestinal loop in the medial and caudal portions of the graft. This variant is used in cases in which the mobilized intestinal segment forms significantly excessive loop in relation to the length of the vascular pedicle. Such situations occur during reconstructive surgeries with the use of the jejunum or the ileum. In case of jejunum, the main reason is the presence of strong, but short vascular trunks, which form effective, but narrow anastomosing arcades. On the other hand, the mesojejunum is relatively short, and the vessels form generally multilayer arcades. Performance of a double resection may help achieve two aims. Firstly, it increases the graft's mobility by resecting the intestinal redundancy in the caudal portion, secondly – it improves blood supply by resecting redundant intestine in the medial portion. Moreover, double resection leads to straightening of the graft, what shortens the passage through the substitutive esophagus, and thus improves its function.

The surgical technique includes parietal ligature and transection of straight vessels, followed by resection of a several-centimeter intestinal segment in the caudal portion of the mobilized graft, and similarly, in the medial portion of the graft, where the intestinal redundancy is most significant, with the continuity of the vascular pedicle left intact. After resection of the redundant intestine in the medial portion of the graft, the remaining stumps should be end-to-end anastomosed (Fig. 3, 4).

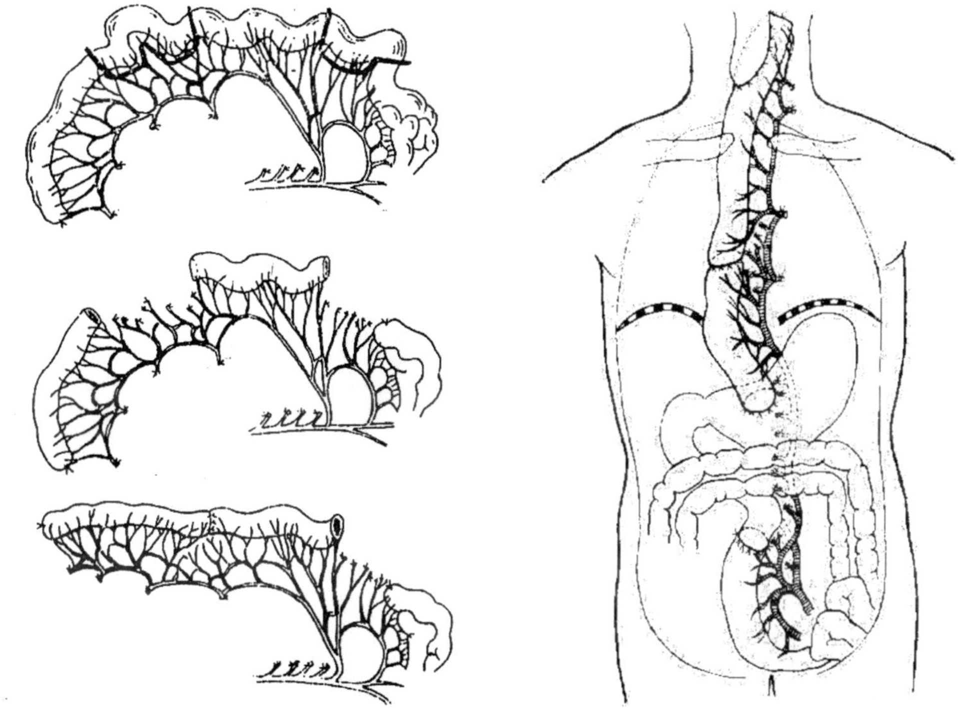

Figure 3 Diagram of double resection of redundant intestine in the medial and caudal portions of the graft

Double resection of redundant intestine is associated with a number of mentioned above advantages. However with inadequate skills of the surgeon, it may result in severe complications in form of insufficiency of anastomosis in the medial portion of the graft.

2. Management of ischaemia in the cephalic portion of the jejunal graft

Insufficiency of vascular arches leads to ischaemia in the cephalic portion of the mobilized graft. This intraoperative complication occurs most commonly in reconstructions using the jejunum. The ischaemic segment of the graft must be resected. Successful completion of a reconstructive surgery seems in such cases impossible. Solution to this difficult situation lies in the knowledge of corrective procedures, which allow to obtain elongation of the graft in the cephalic portion. Presented below are the following techniques of corrective surgery:

- Insertion from the ileum on middle colic vascular pedicle
- Insertion from the colon on ileocolic vascular pedicle

- Insertion from the colon on left colic vascular pedicle
- Secondary mobilization of a pedicled intestinal graft

The choice of a kind of corrective surgery with the use of an insertion is based on an extremely thorough evaluation and analysis of vasculature in the small intestine and the whole colon. An insertion in the cephalic portion of the graft must have its own long vascular pedicle, what will enable adequate elongation of the primary graft and successful termination of the reconstructive surgery.

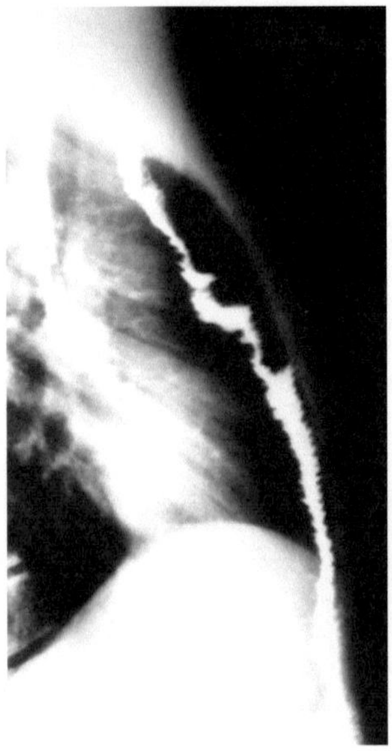

Figure 4 Radiogram of the substitutive esophagus after double resection (lateral projection)

Another way out of the ischemic problem in the cephalic portion of the graft is the method of its secondary mobilization. Secondary mobilization enables elongation of the graft by several centimeters without insertion on another vascular pedicle, what gives a chance to produce a substitutive esophagus on primary vascular pedicle.

2.1 Insertion from the ileum on middle colic vascular pedicle

This variant of corrective surgery should be chosen when there are adequate vascular arrangements between the ileocolic vessels and the vessels in the terminal portion of the ileum, and at the same time the anastomosing arcades between the ileocolic vessels and right and middle colic vessels are broad and effective. Only this kind of vascular anastomosis provides an opportunity to create an insertion on a very long middle colic vascular pedicle.

The surgical technique involves ligating and transecting the ileocolic and right colic vessels and intestinal trunks in the terminal portion of the ileum beyond their ramifications, maintaining the blood flow through the anastomosing arcades. The procedure is associated with the necessity of resecting the caecum and the ascending colon (Fig. 5).

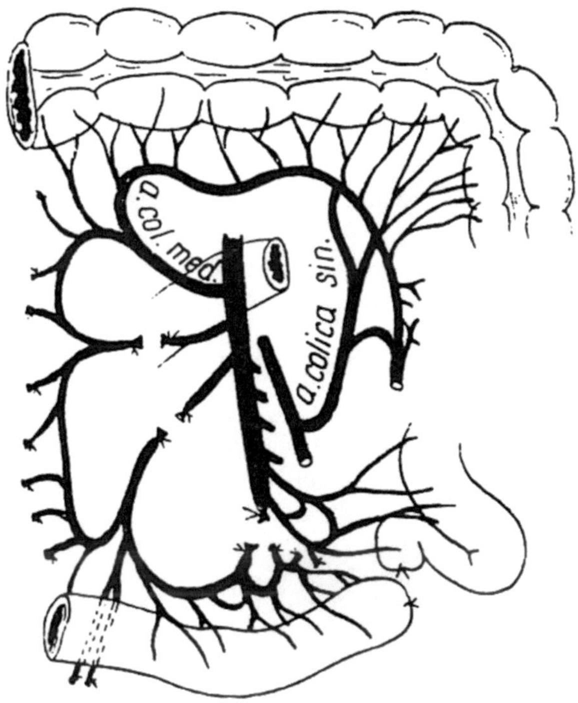

Figure 5 Diagram of mobilization of insertion from the ileum on middle colic vascular pedicle

The next stage includes anastomosing the distal, caudal portion of the primary graft from the jejunum with the insertion made from the ileum. In this way a graft is formed on two independent vascular pedicles consisting in its caudal portion of the jejunum and in the cephalic portion – of the ileum (Fig. 6).

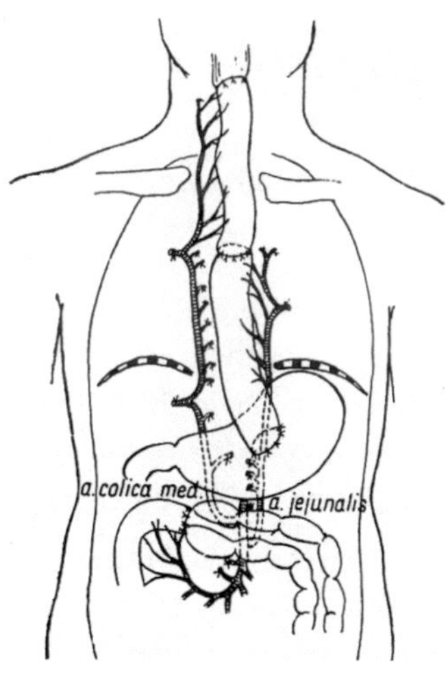

Figure 6 Diagram of double-pedicle substitutive esophagus from the jejunum with an insertion from the ileum on middle colic vascular pedicle

Subsequent stages of the procedure include positioning of the graft in the retrosternal canal, reconstruction of the gastrointestinal tract continuity in the abdomen and anastomosing the graft with the cervical esophagus and the stomach.

A drawback of this type of corrective surgery is that it leaves a relatively large intestinal defect in the abdominal cavity.

However its main advantage is a chance to complete successfully the esophageal reconstruction. Thus the function of the esophagus created in this way, as shown in remote follow up of patients operated on with this method, is very good, what may be attributed to the fact that the whole graft is made from the small intestine with a vivid peristalsis (Fig. 7).

2.2. Insertion from the colon on ileocolic vascular pedicle

If the vasculature in the ileocolic angle is inadequate for a corrective surgery by means of a modality described above, and at the same time anastomoses between the ileocolic and the right and middle colic vessels are long and effective, there are good conditions to produce an insertion from the colon on a long ileocolic vascular pedicle.

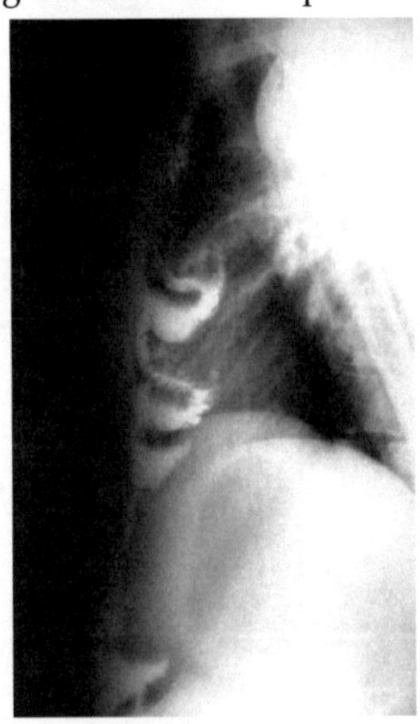

Figure 7 Radiogram of the double-pedicle substitutive esophagus from the jejunum with an insertion from the ileum on middle colic vascular pedicle (lateral projection)

The surgical technique is similar to this described above. After mobilization of the terminal segment of the ileum and the right colon, the graft on ileocolic pedicle should be isolated from the distal segment of the right colon. The right and middle colic vessels are ligated and transected and the caecum and proximal portion of the ascending colon are resected. Thus a graft from the colon on a long ileocolic vascular pedicle is mobilized (Fig. 8).

In the next stage the primary jejunal graft is anastomosed with the insertion produced from the colon. Thus a double-pedicled graft is formed, the caudal portion of which consists of the jejunum, and the cephalic portion – of the colon (Fig. 9).

Subsequent stages of the procedure include positioning of the double-pedicle graft in the retrosternal canal, reconstructing the gastrointestinal tract continuity in the abdomen by anastomosing the ileum with the left part of the transverse colon and anastomosing the graft with the stomach and cervical esophagus.

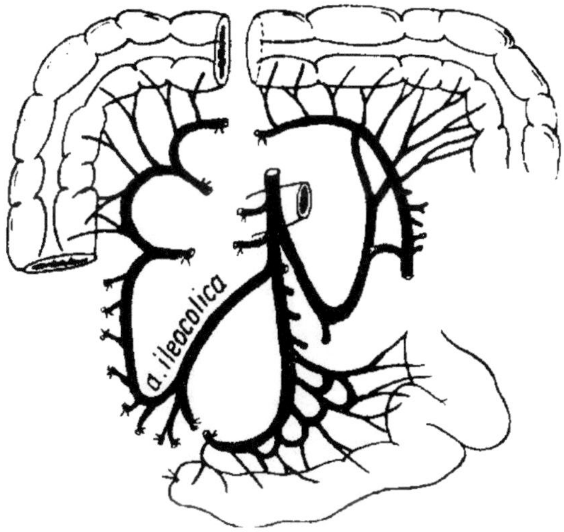

Figure 8 Diagram of mobilization of an insertion from the colon on ileocolic vascular pedicle

It is worth mentioning that insertion from the colon prepared according to this modality is positioned antiperistaltically, and the distal part of the graft made from the jejunum – isoperistaltically.

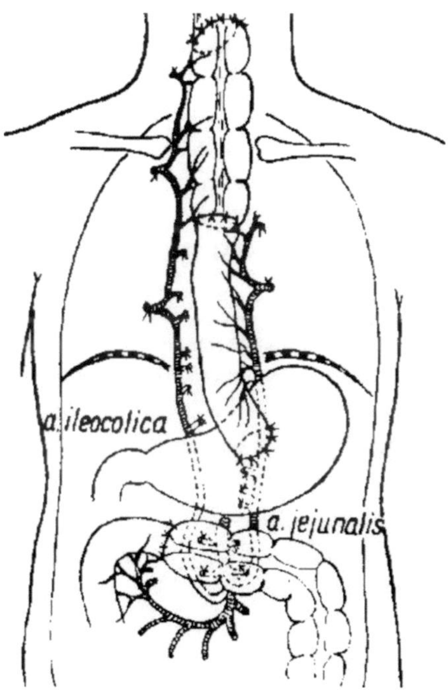

Figure 9 Diagram of a double-pedicle substitutive esophagus from the jejunum with an insertion from the colon on ileocolic vascular pedicle

The main advantage of this variant of corrective surgery is the possibility of completing the reconstructive procedure.

The main disadvantage, similarly as in the first presented variant, is a relatively large intestinal defect in the abdominal cavity.

The function of this substitutive esophagus, as shown in remote examinations of involved patients, is good (Fig. 10).

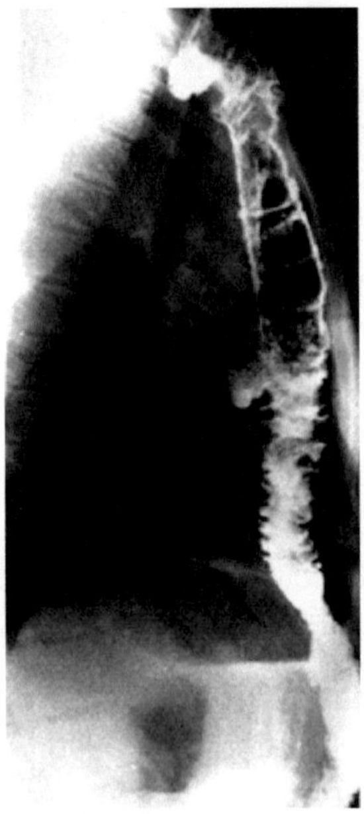

Figure 10 Radiogram of a double-pedicle substitutive esophagus from the jejunum with an insertion from the colon on ileocolic vascular pedicle (lateral projection)

2.3. Insertion from the colon on left colic vascular pedicle

The third variant of corrective surgery involves preparation of an isoperistaltic insertion from the colon on left colic vascular pedicle. This surgical modality is possible when there are exceptionally advantageous vascular arrangements between the right and left colic vessels. In order to enable precise evaluation of vasculature, the right colon and the transverse colon have to be mobilized. Mobilization of the insertion may be undertaken only if the evaluation proves positive. The greater omentum has to be resected. The middle and right colic vessels are ligated and transected. Following transection at an appropriate level of the arch anastomosing the ileocolic and right colic vessels, a segment of the ascending colon, long enough to be used to produce an insertion, has to be isolated. The hepatic flexure of the colon, proximal portion of the transverse colon and the caecum are resected. Thus an isoperistaltic segment of the ascending colon on a long left colic vascular pedicle is isolated (Fig. 11).

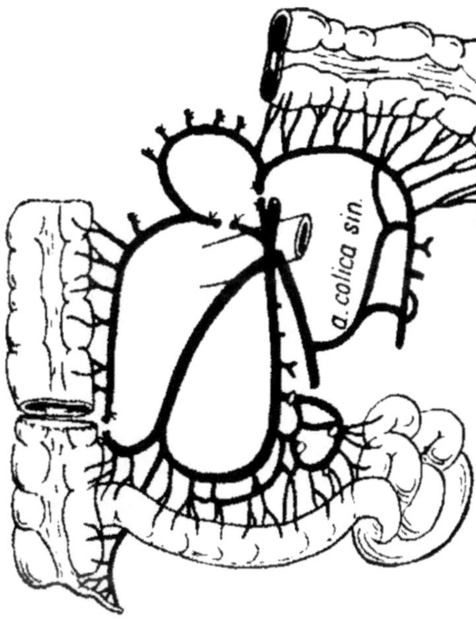

Figure 11 Diagram of mobilization of an insertion from the colon on left colic vascular pedicle

Next the prepared insertion has to be anastomosed with the remaining portion of the primary graft. In this way a double-pedicle graft, consisting from a jejunal segment in the caudal portion, and of an isoperistaltic segment of the colon in the cephalic portion, is produced (Fig. 12).

Subsequent stages of the procedure include positioning of the graft in the retrosternal canal, reconstructing the gastrointestinal tract in the abdomen by anastomosing the ileum with the left transverse colon and anastomosing the graft with the cervical esophagus and the stomach. This variant of surgery, similarly to both previously presented modalities, possesses an important advantage, i.e. the possibility of successful completion of the reconstructive surgery.

A relatively significant intestinal defect in the abdominal cavity is considered to be the main disadvantage.

Remote evaluation of patients operated on according to this modality displayed and efficient function of the esophagus reconstructed in this way (Fig. 13).

Summing up the above presented double-pedicle reconstructions, it should be emphasized that they belong to extremely complicated techniques and require perfect mastering of the surgical technique as well as enormous experience of the surgeon. And it should be emphasized again that the modalities are original and unique modifications of the reconstructive surgeries, which enable successful completion of the surgery.

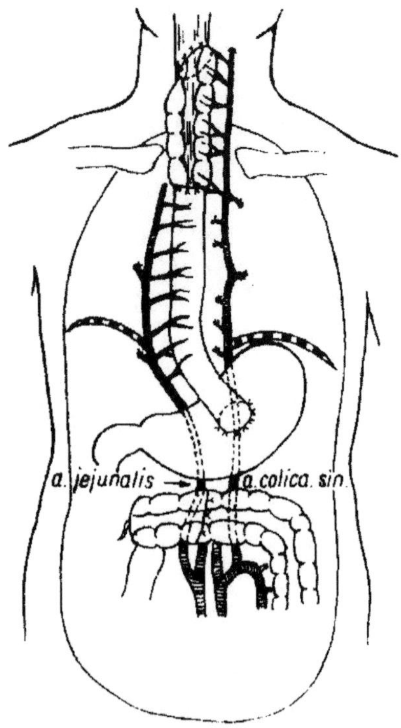

Figure 12 Diagram of a double-pedicle substitutive esophagus from the jejunum with an insertion from the colon on left colic vascular pedicle

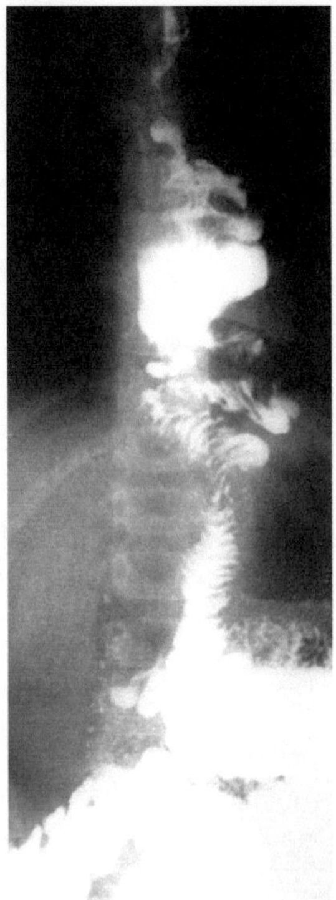

Figure 13 Radiogram of a double-pedicle substitutive esophagus from the jejunum with an insertion from the colon on left colic vascular pedicle (A-P projection)

2.4. Secondary mobilization of the graft

Another original solution, which extends the possibility of using the jejunum to create a substitutive esophagus and enables a successful termination of reconstructive surgery involves secondary mobilization of the pedicled graft, proposed and used in esophageal reconstructions by Bernat in 1980.

The below presented modality is especially useful in cases in which the mobilized jejunal graft appears too short to be anastomosed with the cervical esophagus.

Excessive stretching and tension in the vascular pedicle of a too short graft lead to narrowing or even obstruction of a lumen in the apex of vascular arches in so-called critical points, what results in ischaemia of the graft and subsequently leads to necrosis (Fig. 14).

A possible solution to this difficult situation may include elongation of a too short graft by one of the means described above, i.e. by means of an insertion from the ileum or the colon on a long vascular pedicle. Another solution, less complicated than production of an insertion on a separate vascular pedicle, is secondary mobilization of the graft according to Bernat.

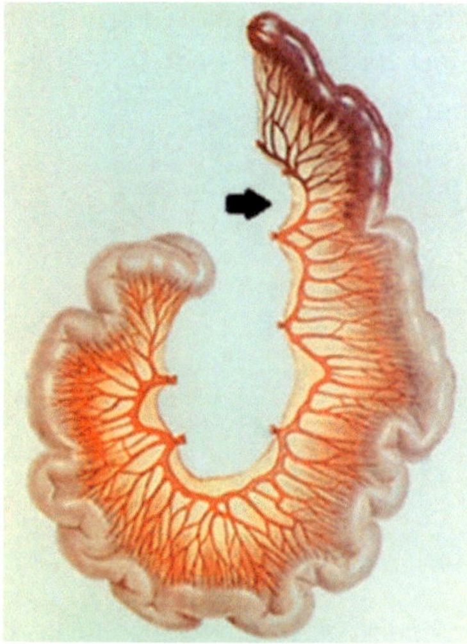

Figure 14 Diagram of a pedicled graft from the jejunum with ischaemia in the cephalic portion of the apex of the vascular arch (arrow)

The method of secondary mobilization involves placement of a too short graft in the presternal subcutaneous canal for several weeks. For this reason the jejunal graft mobilized on a vascular pedicle should be translocated beyond the colon and beyond the stomach to the epigastrium. The distal, caudal segment of the graft should be anastomosed to the stomach, and the proximal, cephalic segment – closed in a cul-de-sack manner. Subsequently, a subcutaneous, presternal canal is formed and the graft is placed in it. Gastric fistula, performed as the first stage prior to the esophageal reconstruction, or during the procedure, allows full nutrition of the patient in the postoperative period (Fig. 15).

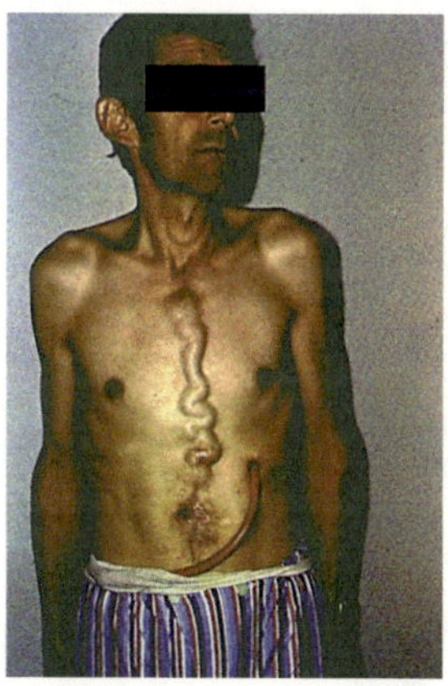

Figure 15 Picture of a patient with a graft temporarily placed in the presternal subcutaneous canal. Gastrostomy drainage visible in the left hypochondrium

The next stage of the surgery may be undertaken after 4-5 weeks, and it includes mobilization of the graft from the subcutaneous canal and placement in the retrosternal canal. The presternal canal is opened with a skin incision above the sternum and continuing to the epigastrium and next the graft together with its vascular pedicle is prepared gently up to the level of the graft's anastomosis to the stomach (Fig. 16).

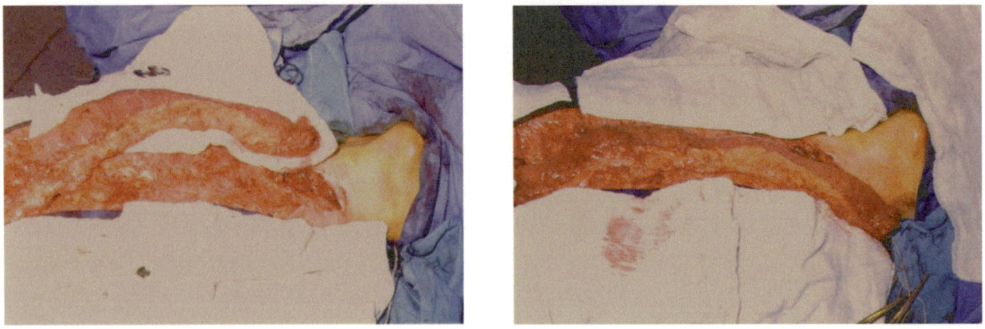

Figure 16 Intraoperative picture of mobilization of the graft from the presternal subcutaneous canal. The elongated graft reaches high up the neck to the level of the mandibular angle.

Next the retrosternal canal is created according to the method described in previous chapters. The mobilized graft is passed in the retrosternal canal and anastomosed to the cervical esophagus.

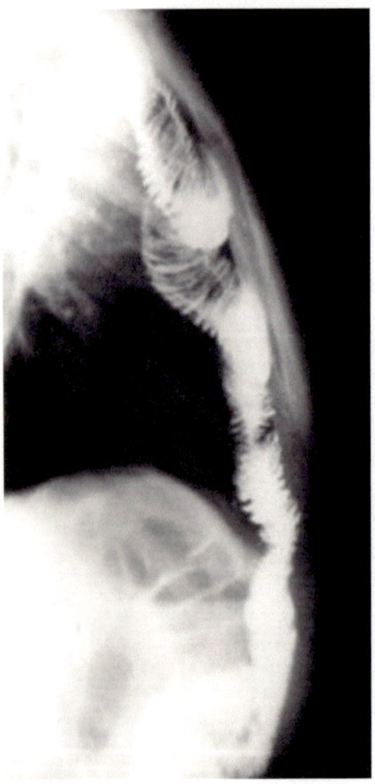

Figure 17 Radiogram of a substitutive esophagus from the jejunum after secondary mobilization (lateral projection)

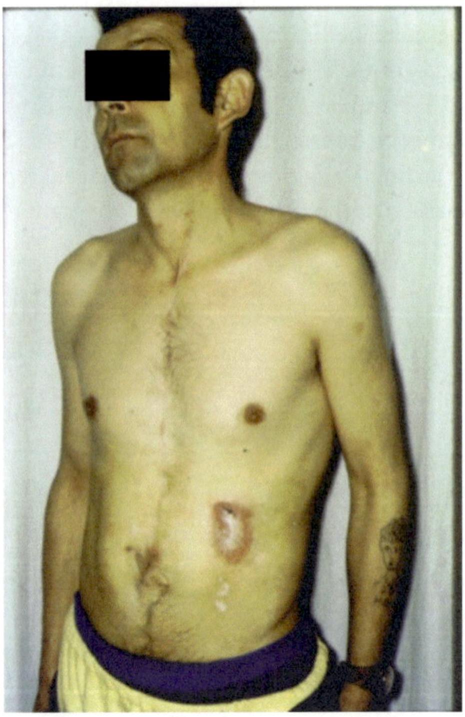

Figure 18 Picture of a patient after completed esophageal reconstruction by means of secondary mobilization of the graft

The advantages of the presented modality include elongation of the graft placed for few weeks in the subcutaneous canal, after secondary mobilization even by 6-7 cm, strengthening of the vascular pedicle, as well as broadening and strengthening of anastomosing arcades. Thus secondary mobilization leads to elongation of the graft and improvement of blood supply, what gives chance for successful termination of the reconstructive surgery.

The only disadvantage of the modality is that the surgical procedure is prolonged by several weeks.

Using this modality, it is possible to achieve a very good final outcome, what was confirmed in postoperative follow up (Fig. 17, 18).

Recapitulating the chapter on complex esophageal reconstructions, it should be emphasized that they belong to highly specialist procedures and should be undertaken by centres with highly educated and trained surgical staff. The main desire of a surgeon is not only to create a substitutive esophagus, but also to attain function of the newly created esophagus most closely resembling this of a natural esophagus. Being aware of this, and having expert knowledge and skills, the surgeon should always strive to choose optimal surgical modality in every single case.

3. References

[1] Jezioro Z. Formation of esophagus from jejunum using own method. I. Segmental excision of excess of mobilized jejunum. Pol Przegl Chir 1973, 45: 1253-1261.

[2] Francioni F, De Giacomo T, Jo Filice M, Anile M, Diso D, Venuta F, Coloni GF. Surgical treatment of redundancy after retrosternal esophagocoloplasty. Minerva Chir 2009, 64: 317-319.

[3] Jezioro Z. Esophagoplasty using the ileum and cecum and insertion of the large intestine on a common ileo-colonic vascular peduncle. Pol Przegl Chir 1966, 38: 455-459.

[4] Jezioro Z. Esophagoplasty with the use of the large intestine, pedunculated on the vasa colica sinistra and with insertion made of the ileum and cecum. Pol Przegl Chir1967, 39: 809-816.

[5] Jezioro Z. Formation of esophagus from jejunum using own method. II. Surgical procedures in cases of insufficiency of vascular arches of the mobilized jejunum. Pol Przegl Chir 1973, 45: 1263-1270.

[6] Bernat M. Total plastic surgery of the retrosternal esophagus with its replacement with jejunum and secondary translocation of the graft using the Jezioro method. Pol Przegl Chir 1977, 49: 19-24.

[7] Bernat M. Formation of complete retrosternal esophagus from the jejunum in cases of cicatricial stenosis of the esophagus and distal part of the stomach by means of secondary shifting of the graft. Pol Przegl Chir 1980, 52: 533-537.

[8] Bernat M, Bader O, Milnerowicz S, Grabowski K, Rosinska T, Blaszczuk J. Colon or ileum for reconstruction of the total esophagus with reference to vascularization. Zentralbl Chir 1985, 110: 1297-1303.

[9] Mansour KA, Bryan FC, Carlson GW. Bowel interposition for esophageal replacement: twenty-five-year experience. Ann Thorac Surg 1997, 64: 752-756.

[10] Nienartowicz M, Strutyńska-Karpińska M, Śliwa B. A novel method of reconstructive surgery of the esophagus. Adv Clin Exp Med 2008, 17: 583-585.

[11] Poh M, Selber JC, Skoracki R, Walsh GL, Yu P. Technical challenges of total esophageal reconstruction using a supercharged jejunal flap. Ann Surg 2011, 253: 1122-1129.

[12] Maurer SV, Estremadoyro V, Reinberg O. Evaluation of an antireflux procedure for colonic interposition in pediatric esophageal replacements. J Pediatr Surg 2011, 46: 594-600.

[13] Oki M, Asato H, Suzuki Y, Umekawa K, Takushima A, Okazaki M, Harii K. Salvage reconstruction of the oesophagus: a retrospective study of 15 cases. J Plast Reconstr Aesthet Surg 2010, 63: 589-597.

[14] Numajiri T, Fujiwara T, Nishino K, Sowa Y, Uenaka M, Masuda S, Fujiwara H, Nakai S, Hisa Y. Double vascular anastomosis for safer free jejunal transfer in unfavorable conditions. J Reconstr Microsurg 2008, 24: 531-536.

[15] Takushima A, Momosawa A, Asato H, Aiba E, Harii K. Double vascular pedicled free jejunum transfer for total esophageal reconstruction. J Reconstr Microsurg 2005, 21: 5-10.

[16] Omura K, Urayama H, Kanehira E, Kaito K, Ohta K, Ishida Y, Takizawa M, Sumitomo H, Watanabe Y. Reconstruction of the thoracic esophagus using jejunal pedicle with vascular anastomoses. J Surg Oncol 2000, 75: 217-219.

[17] YasudaT, Shiozaki H. Esophageal reconstruction with colon tissue. Surg Today 2011, 41: 745-753.

[18] Mogos D, Vasile I, Paun I, Florescu M, Valcea D, Dumitrelea D, Ungureanu G, Nedelcuta C. Esophagoplasty with right ileocolon, technical problems. Chirurgia (Bukur) 2000, 95: 79-84.

[19] Okazaki M, Asato H, Takushima A, Nakatsuka T, Ueda K. Secondary reconstruction of failed esophageal reconstruction. Ann Plast Surg 2005, 54: 530-537.

[20] Randjelovic T, Dikic S, Filipovic B, Gacic D, Bilanovic D, Stanisavljevic N. Short-segment jejunoplasty: the option treatment in the management of benign esophageal stricture. Dis Esophagus 2007, 20: 239-246.

[21] Inoue Y, Tai Y, Fujita H, Tanaka S, Migita H, Kiyokawa K, Hirano M, Kakegawa T. A retrospective study of 66 esophageal reconstructions using microvascular anastomoses: problems and our methods for atypical cases. Plast Reconstr Surg 1994, 94: 277-284.

Chapter 4

Diagnosis and Treatment of Postoperative Complications After Esophageal Reconstruction with Pedicled Intestinal Segments

Esophageal reconstructions belong to complicated and extensive surgical procedures burdened with a significant percentage of postoperative complications. The complications can be divided into two groups. The first group includes complications arising during mobilization of the graft or immediately in the perioperative period and are referred to as early or perisurgical complications. The latter develop long time after the operation and may be considered so-called disorders of the esophageal substitute.

According to literature, the prevalence of early complications ranges from 3.6% to 16%. The number of late complications is significantly higher. According to some authors, very good or good function of the esophageal substitute may be achieved in about 50–65% of patients.

1. Early complications after esophageal reconstruction

1.1. Necrosis of a part or a whole intestinal graft

Complications of this type may develop both, during the operation as well as in the perioperative period. They occur intraoperatively in cases in which assessment of the vascular system in the intestinal segment designated for the graft has been wrong prior to the graft mobilization. At this stage of the surgery, i.e. during evaluation of the type of vasculature and its adequacy, haste is inadvisable, especially that definitely favourable vascular arrangements within the small intestine mesentery occur in 30-40% of population, while definitely unfavourable arrangements are observed in further 30%. The remaining patients have intermediary types, which may prove most difficult to evaluate. For this reason in order to enable more precise assessment of the adequacy of blood supply to the intestinal segment designated for the pedicled esophageal graft, ultrasound Doppler examinations are performed intraoperatively. And even these additional possibilities of evaluating adequacy of circulation do not reduce to the minimum the risk of complications in the form of graft ischaemia. It should be remembered that in sustaining vitality of the mobilized intestinal graft also the venous system plays equally important role. Some authors even believe it is of primary significance. Definite, acute ischaemia of the graft, or definite disturbances in the venous outflow can be diagnosed easily. In case of the former, i.e. acute arterial ischaemia the symptoms are extremely tempestuous and difficult to be overlooked. Acute ischaemia manifests itself in the form of lack of pulsation in the distal straight vessels of the investigated intestinal segment, its pallor, sometimes marble-like appearance of the wall and its cooling. At the same time veins in such cases are evidently less filled with blood. In case of disturbances in the venous outflow with maintained arterial blood flow, the investigated intestinal segment becomes cyanosed with an evident venous overfilling and stasis, progressive oedema and increased peristalsis in the investigated intestinal segment. However when occlusion of venous outflow is incomplete, the symptoms are definitely less evident, as the wall is slightly cyanosed, sometimes reversibly, and oedema of the wall is almost invisible. The disturbances, very difficult to evaluate, are extremely dangerous, as, like in case of arterial ischemia, lead to necrosis of the graft, while definite clinical symptoms appear few days after initially seemingly normal postoperative course. For this reason some surgical centres perform almost as a routine mobilization of the jejunal graft accompanied by additional vascular anastomoses to support blood supply to the graft. Implementation of this procedure, which improves blood supply, has significantly reduced the number of complications associated with ischemia.

Disturbances in blood supply to the intestinal segment may also occur at further stages of the operation. One of the most significant and very important surgical procedure is to form the retrosternal canal and pass the mobilized graft through the canal onto the neck. The procedure may seem relatively simple. However our clinical experience points to various hazards associated with this stage, including those concerning blood supply to the intestinal segment to be passed through the canal. Due to anatomical conditions in the mediastinum the superior opening of the retrosternal canal from the side of the neck, at the level of the jugular notch of the sternum, is significantly narrower in comparison to the inferior opening from the side of the abdomen. That is why the graft is most exposed to pressure in the superior opening of the canal, just beyond the left sternoclavicular joint, what may contribute to ischemia in the cephalic portion of the graft and its necrosis. For these reasons the superior opening of the retrosternal canal has to be broad enough, both in the frontal as well as in the sagittal planes, to accommodate the intestinal graft together with its mesentery without any pressure. Some surgical centres, as mentioned in previous chapters, remove the left sternoclavicular joint in order to form at this level an adequately broad retrosternal canal. On the other hand, formation of an adequately broad retrosternal canal at the level of inferior entrance, i.e. from the side of the abdomen, in many cases requires radial incision of the diaphragm, sagitally in the canal axis, what successfully broadens the entrance and prevents any pressure exerted possibly by the diaphragm on the graft's pedicle in the retrosternal canal.

Another hazard to the graft's vitality and development of its ischaemia is associated with intestinal torsion around the vascular pedicle in the retrosternal canal, what may easily happen in cases of reconstruction with the ileum or the jejunum, when, in view of the anatomy of the vascular systems, there is a significant excess of the intestine in relation to its mesentery. For this reason passing the graft through the retrosternal canal must be performed extremely gently, and in case of any disturbances in blood supply to the graft, the situation has to be immediately revised and diagnosed, and next removed. Only normally supplied graft authorizes continuation of the operation.

In the perioperative period the main clinical symptoms of the graft's necrosis include pain in the neck and behind the sternum. The symptoms are accompanied by dyspnoea, increased body temperature, accelerated pulse and discharge of blood or brownish matter through the gastric fistula. Physical examination reveals inflammatory oedema with evident tenderness to palpation in the region of the cervical wound. Also the epigastric region is tender to palpation, and when the symptoms of necrosis are fully developed, the symptoms of peritonitis set in. Accessory investigations, especially chest x-ray reveal evident widening of the mediastinal shadow, and sometimes presence of exudate in the pleural cavity (Fig. 1).

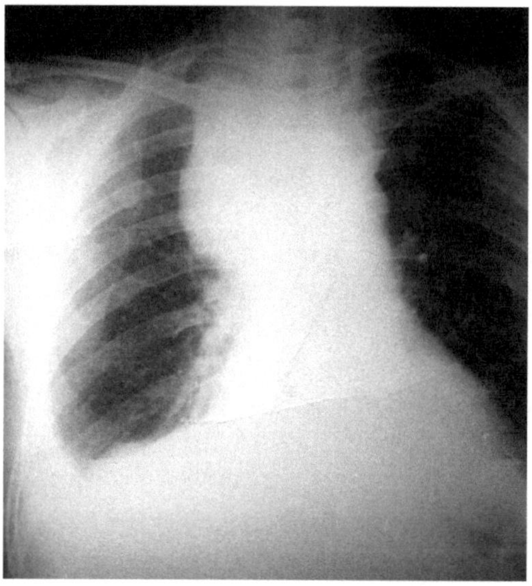

Figure 1 Radiogram of patient's chest with necrosis of the graft (A-P projection). Visible significant dilatation of the mediastinum and exudate in the right pleural cavity

The management of choice is a repeated operation – removal of the necrotic graft, mediastinal and peritoneal drainage, formation of a salivary fistula in the cervical esophagus, management of the opening in the stomach after removed graft and formation of a decompressing gastric fistula, if it was not placed before to feed the patient.

In case of ischaemia and necrosis of the cephalic portion of the graft alone, the clinical symptoms are limited to changes in the neck and inflammatory conditions in the mediastinum occur rarely. The surgical management in such cases is limited to removal of necrotic cephalic portion of the graft, with maintained healthy portion closed in a cul-de–sac manner in the cephalic part, since it may prove useful later on for reparative surgery. Thus prepared remaining segment of the graft has to be placed in the abdominal cavity. Such procedures as formation of a salivary fistula on the neck, drainage of the neck and superior opening to the retrosternal canal as well as decompression of the gastric fistula give chance to save the patient's life. A reparative operation, which consists for example in elongation of the remaining primary graft with another, pedicled or free intestinal graft, may be undertaken at a later stage. Reparative operations of this type are especially complicated procedures and should be performed in highly specialized centres with a significant experience in this field.

Disruption of the graft's pedicle is another, extremely rare complication. This situation may occur during incompetent pulling of the graft through the retrosternal canal, when, after termination of pulling, when the intestine appears in the superior opening of the retrosternal canal, in order to place it higher up in the cephalic direction, the graft is pulled not by the intestine, but by the pedicle. This fatal complication destroys the graft's vitality practically irreversibly and in principle cannot occur during reconstructive procedure. However, should this situation occur, the damaged graft has to be removed and replaced by another graft mobilized from another intestinal segment.

1.2. Pneumothorax

Another complication, which is associated directly with the performed operation at the stage of formation of the retrosternal canal, is pleural injury and opening of the pleural cavity. During creation of the retrosternal canal it should be remembered that the right and the left mediastinal pleura approach and adhere to each other at the level of the III and IV costal cartilage. The right pleura is often found not in the midline, but it deviates to the left. Thus on creation of the retrosternal canal, especially at the stage of widening of the canal to the sides, there is a risk of pleural injury and opening of the pleural cavity, most commonly on the right side. Pneumothorax, if noticed, in principle does not pose an immediate life-threatening danger. A small opening in the pleura may be sealed quickly by immediate passing of the graft through the retrosternal canal. But it should be remembered that prior to termination of the operation and removal of the endotracheal tube the thorax should be punctured and the lung should be decompressed. Chest x-ray is mandatory immediately following the operation.

Complications may sporadically occur as a result of minor pleural injuries in the perioperative period. On the other hand, long time after the surgery even small pleural injury may lead to the formation of pleural hernia in the esophageal substitute, what will be discussed in subsequent chapters of the review.

1.3. Insufficiency of cervical anastomosis

Complication in the form of insufficient cervical anastomosis occurs rarely. Excluding errors of a technical nature during cervical anastomosis, the complication may occur basically for two reasons. Firstly, whet the intestinal graft in the cephalic portion is poorly vascularized. Secondly, when the cervical anastomosis was performed under significant tension, what usually occurs when the mobilized and pulled through the retrosternal canal graft appears too short.

Clinical findings include inflammatory infiltration on the neck with the presence of salivary fistula. Surgical intervention consists in drainage in the region of the cervical anastomosis and superior entrance to the retrosternal canal. The patient should be nourished through a gastric fistula until healing of the infiltration. Permanent spitting out of the saliva and oral washes with antiseptic solutions provide additionally good effect. Reconstruction of the cervical anastomosis should be considered after healing of the inflammatory condition.

1.4. Salivary fistula in the region of cervical anastomosis

Salivary fistulas belong to most common complications associated with esophageal reconstruction. In majority of cases they do not require repeating of the operation and heal as a result of conservative treatment. However in case of a fistula, after its healing a cicatrical stenosis of the cervical anastomosis may occur, which may be troublesome for the patient on oral feeding, and on many occasion necessitates a reoperation, which in many cases may prove more difficult than the whole reconstructive surgery (Fig. 2).

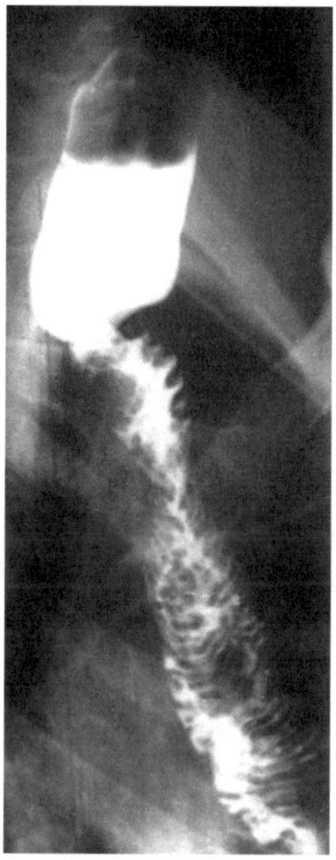

Figure 2 Radiogram of esophageal substitute from the jejunum (oblique projection). Visible anastomotic cervical stenosis after healed fistula

Review of literature on the problem demonstrates explicitly that cervical anastomotic fistulas are significantly more commonly observed after reconstructions with the colon than after operations with the use of the small intestine. Numerous authors see the reasons for this condition in a lack of peristalsis in the colon graft, inadequate lumen between the cervical esophagus and the colon, and, additionally, the presence of bacterial flora in the colon, what provides favourable conditions for the development of a fistula, in contrast to reconstructions with the small intestine, which are characterized by vivid peristalsis, lumen comparable to the esophagus as well as bacterial flora different than in the colon. Moreover, opinion of the authors who see the reasons for development of cervical anastomotic fistulas in insufficient blood supply to the region of the anastomosis, e.g. as a result of thrombi in small veins, seems highly justified.

The clinical image of a cervical anastomotic fistula is relatively characteristic and does not pose any diagnostic problems. The fistula usually manifests itself about 6-7 days after the surgery. A limited, not very diffuse inflammatory infiltration appears in the region of the wound scar, often similar to those which may be observed in non-healed subcutaneous ligatures. On opening of the infiltration there is visible salivary leakage. The patient usually does not report any complaints at this time. Oral administration of a small amount of boiled water stained with methylene blue reveals leakage of the stain and saliva through the fistula to the dressing. Another method to confirm the presence of a cervical fistula is to administer orally aqueous solution of a contrast medium and x-ray the patient. However if the fistula is small, it is not always demonstrated on radiological examination, although the presence of a fistula is certain clinically. In conservative treatment, apart from changing dressings several times a day, it is most important to exclude feeding by mouth, constant spitting out saliva and washing the oral cavity with antiseptic solutions several times a day and always before the night. In this time the patient is nourished through a gastric fistula.

1.5. Injury of the recurrent laryngeal nerve

Injury of the recurrent laryngeal nerve belongs to relatively rare complications and affects about 6% of the operated patients. It occurs during preparation and isolation of the cervical esophagus prior to cervical anastomosis with the graft and is most commonly associated with brutal manipulations in the region of the nerve. In order to avoid this complication, far reaching care and delicacy during performance of the cervical stage of the reconstructive surgery are highly recommended.

Injury of the recurrent laryngeal nerve manifests itself in the form of hoarseness, and laryngological examination reveals vocal cord paralysis on the side of injured nerve. As mentioned above, the complication is not severe and does not impair in a significant way the function of the esophageal substitute.

2. Diagnosis and treatment of late complications after esophageal reconstructions

Long-term complications after esophageal reconstructions may be divided into two main groups. The first group includes these complications which impair the basic function of the esophageal substitute; the latter encompasses so-called disorders of the esophageal substitutes, which, in principle, may be mainly attributed to conditions and disorders associated with gastric, and often biliary reflux to the esophageal substitute. The new esophageal substitute created from a segment of the small intestine or colon, is not equipped with adequate defense mechanisms as a natural esophagus. Rare diseases of esophageal substitutes, such as malignant tumours, which may occur 20-30 years after the reconstructive surgery, constitute a separate group of rare conditions and are described in literature as single case reports.

In the opinion of various surgical centres, very good or good function of the esophageal substitutes is reported in about 50-65% of the patients. The remaining cases are affected by various disorders and/or diseases of the esophageal substitutes, which significantly impair the quality of feeding. The changes often pose significant diagnostic difficulties and on many occasions require complicated repair procedures.

The diagnosis of disorders of the esophageal substitutes is not easy, the more that the possibilities of accessory investigations are to some extent limited mainly due to topographic changes associated with the reconstructive procedure. For this reason it seems justifiable to present in this place the diagnostic possibilities in patients after esophageal reconstructions.

2.1. Diagnosis of the esophageal substitute

Radiological examinations

The diagnosis of the esophageal substitute is not easy, and the scope of diagnostic procedures is limited. For many years, prior to the introduction of endoscopic procedures, accessory investigations after esophageal reconstructions were limited only to radiological assessment with the use of contrast medium and laboratory tests evaluating function of the esophageal substitute on the basis of possible disturbances in the absorption of basic substances, like proteins, lipids, carbohydrates, vitamins, etc.

However radiological examinations, which present a definite image as far as the passage through the esophageal substitute is concerned, do not allow precise diagnosis and evaluation of certain disorders of the esophageal substitutes, such as for example inflammatory conditions associated with reflux. The role of endoscopy cannot be overestimated in this respect, as it not only enables diagnosis of inflammatory conditions, but also informs about their severity and provides many other opportunities, which will be discussed in further chapters devoted to disorders of the esophageal substitutes and their treatment. Despite the above-mentioned advantages and benefits associated with the introduction of endoscopic methods to the diagnosis of disorders of the esophageal substitutes, the role of radiological examinations is still valuable. Radiological examinations remain an indispensable tool in the diagnosis of many cases and many disorders, such as for example pleural hernia, or examinations evaluating passage through the esophageal substitute. And although the latter cases, i.e. passage of food through the esophageal substitute may be evaluated by means of isotope examination, they are less frequently used due to significant costs. Other radiological methods include computerized tomography and magnetic resonance. Apart from high costs of the examinations, both diagnostic methods are not always specific and tender enough in relation to changes which may occur in the esophageal substitute. On the other hand, endocavital ultrasound evaluation seems to reveal new diagnostic possibilities, as it allows evaluation of changes in the walls of the investigated organs.

Endoscopy of the esophageal substitute

The endoscopic technique is difficult, what is associated with the topography of the esophageal substitute in the anterior mediastinum. Such a position of the graft requires forward relocation of the cervical segment of the esophagus from the prevertebral space towards the anterior mediastinum in order to enable anastomosis with the graft. Cervical end-side-to-side anastomosis with the throat or cervical esophagus is advantageous in this respect that the anastomosis lumen is relatively wide and even in case of complications in the form of salivary fistula, after healing the anastomotic stenosis is uncommon. However this type of cervical anastomosis, together with a new position of the cervical portion of natural esophagus contribute to a difficult passage from the throat to the portion reconstructed with the intestinal segment and further, to distal part of the esophageal substitute on endoscopic examination. The endoscope has to turn twice at the angle of 70^0 on a short distance. The first turn is necessary to pass through the cervical anastomosis, the second – after getting through the cervical anastomosis, i.e. on passage from the prevertebral space on the neck to the anterior mediastinum, i.e. the retrosternal canal (Fig. 3). Another difficulty in this region is associated with an osteoarticular limitation – the left sternoclavicular joint. After passing the endoscope through this segment and its insertion to the esophageal substitute in the retrosternal canal, it should be remembered that in many cases, especially after reconstructions with the jejunum or ileum, the esophageal substitute in this region is quite tortuous, what poses additional difficulties on endoscopic evaluation. Another drawback on endoscopy is connected with immobilization of the tortuous course intestine by numerous adhesions to the surrounding tissues, what significantly hampers the examination and does not allow straightening of the intestine. Thus, undertaking a trial to evaluate the esophageal substitute by means of endoscopic examination, the endoscopist has to be aware of all the difficulties and hazards associated with the unskillful performance of the procedure. Endoscopic examination should be performed by an endoscopist with high expertise. Moreover, good knowledge of technical details of various types of esophageal reconstruction, which facilitates maneuvering in topographic conditions which had been changes during the operation is mandatory.

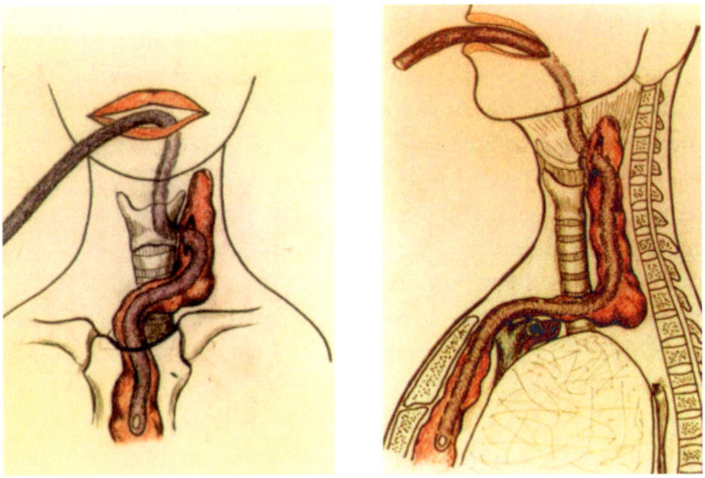

Figure 3 Endoscopy of the esophageal substitute (A-P and lateral projection)

Introduction of endoscopic technique to evaluation of the esophageal substitute opens a number of both, diagnostic and therapeutic possibilities. Endoscopy provides opportunity to evaluate the esophageal substitute, possible changes within the mucous membrane and their severity. It also evaluates the function of the stomach, the efficacy of its emptying and the presence of gastric or biliary reflux to the esophageal lumen. Moreover, it enables detection and treatment of changes originating in the esophageal substitute many years after the reconstructive procedure. Thanks to endoscopic technique, it possible in many cases to make proper diagnosis, when other accessory investigations fail.

The advantage of endoscopy lies not only in the fact that it enables an exact diagnosis, but it also allows implementing adequate therapy. This concerns bleedings, which may be controlled by means of endoscopic methods, or the presence of polyps in the esophageal substitute, which may be removed endoscopically. Thus the above-mentioned endoscopic methods permit more exact diagnosis and, in many cases, treatment of esophageal substitutes without the necessity of complicated repair procedures.

2.2. Late complications in the region of cervical anastomosis

Abnormal functioning of the esophageal substitute may be affected by a number of factors. Among them, the decisive role is played by the type of cervical anastomosis. In the reconstructive surgery of the esophagus an end-to-end anastomosis is most commonly employed. The side-to-side, or end-to-side anastomoses also find their place, but they are used rarely and are reserved for selected cases. However in our experience, an end-side-to-side anastomosis, also referred to as an "oblique" type, allows to attain sufficient diameter of the cervical anastomosis and thus gives a better functional outcome.

2.2.1 Cicatrical stenosis of the cervical anastomosis

Cicatrical stenosis of the cervical anastomosis is the most common complication occurring long time after the reconstructive procedure. It is usually preceded by the presence of even a small fistula in the region of cervical anastomosis, which, after healing contributes to formation of a cicatrical stenosis. The above complication is observed definitely more often after an end-to-end anastomosis and after reconstructions with the use of a pedicled colon segment. As mentioned before, the reason for this complication is sought in a diverse physiology of the colon in comparison to the small intestine, as well as in an even slight ischaemia at the site of the anastomosis.

Depending on the degree of the anastomotic stenosis, the patient may experience more or less pronounced difficulties on swallowing. Radiological examination reveals narrowing of the cervical anastomosis, often with evident dilatation of the cervical esophagus before the anastomosis and retention of the contrast medium (Fig. 4, 5). In, luckily, few cases an almost complete cicatrical occlussion of the anastomosis may develop, what is associated with an additional hazard in the form of aspiration pneumonia. The patient in such a case complains of a troublesome necessity of constant spitting out saliva which accumulates in the mouth, and at night choking may often occur, leading to respiratory infections (Fig. 6).

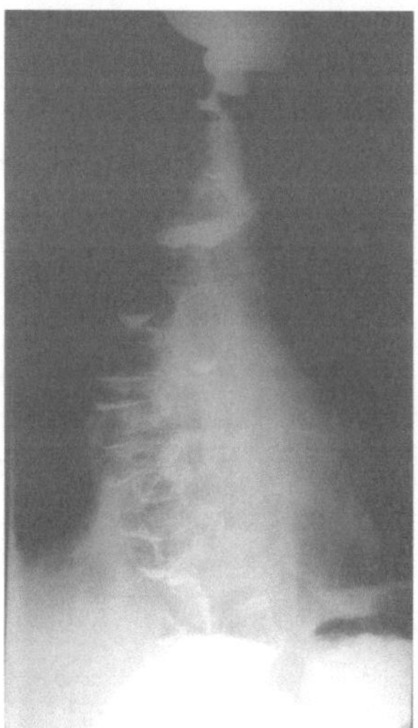

Figure 4 Radiogram of esophageal substitute from the colon (A-P projection). Visible cicatrical stenosis of the cervical anastomosis after healed fistula

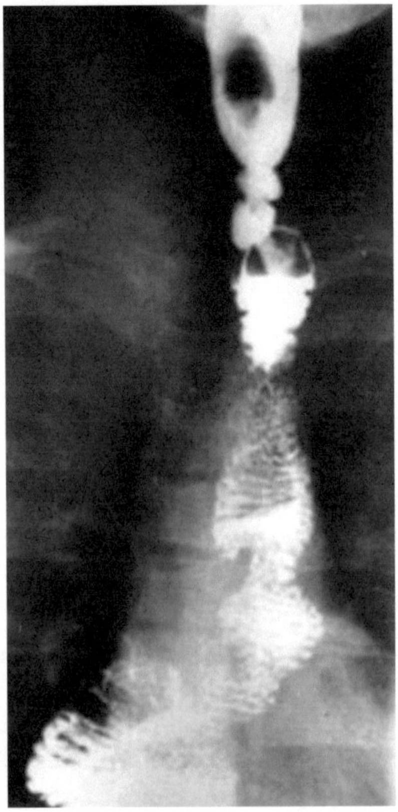

Figure 5 Radiogram of esophageal substitute from the jejunum (A-P projection). Visible cicatrical stenosis of the cervical anastomosis after healed fistula

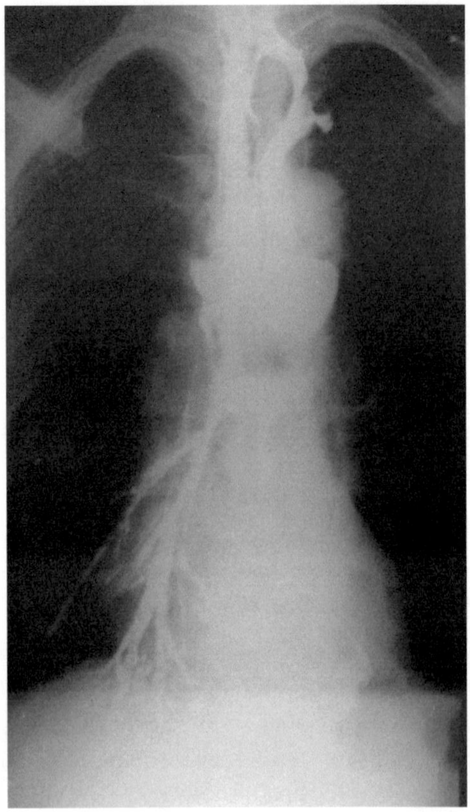

Figure 6 Radiogram of a significant stenosis of cervical anastomosis after esophageal reconstruction with the colon (A-P projection, examination with aqueous solution of contrast medium). The patient chokes. Bronchial tree filled with contrast medium

In case of less extensive stenoses, a good outcome may be achieved by means of an endoscopic dilatation. This usually requires several sessions, during which the stenosis is dilated until a desired diameter is obtained, i.e. about 15 mm. On the other hand, if the cicatrical anastomotic stenoses are extensive, repair procedures: reconstruction of the anastomosis (reanastomosis), or bypassing are necessary. The final decision as to the reconstructive technology is made during the procedure in relation to the intraoperatively observed local conditions at the site of the anastomosis. It is worth noting that the procedures, seemingly easy, may pose many technical problems, starting from difficulties in preparation of a segment of the cervical esophagus and the cephalic portion of the esophageal substitute, with the vascular pedicle as its most important element, which usually adheres most to the surrounding tissues. Destruction of the vascular pedicle in this region results in a loss of the cephalic segment of the esophageal substitute due to lack of blood supply. Further difficulties are associated with repeated cervical anastomosing. It should be remembered that both, the cervical portion of the esophagus, and primarily the cephalic portion of the esophageal substitute are difficult to mobilize, and often so firmly fixed with adhesions, that they become practically impossible to mobilize. Thus sometimes the repair operation in this region may exceed in difficulty the whole reconstructive procedure. According to experience, any repair procedures on esophageal substitutes should be performed in specialist centres with high level of expertise in this matter, as damage inflicted by improper conduct of the procedure may prove difficult to repair even in a specialist centre.

2.2.2. Diverticula in the region of cervical anastomosis

Diverticula in the region of cervical anastomosis are often observed after an end-to-side, or end-side-to-side anastomoses. They usually occur when too long, blind intestinal stump is left in the region of the anastomosis. Initially after the surgery the complaints are almost imperceptible for the patient, however with time the diverticulum enlarges, fills with saliva and food and, exerting pressure on the cervical anastomosis, may significantly impair the act of swallowing. The condition becomes especially important after reconstructions with the colon, when active peristalsis is absent, and the swallowed food passes downwards driven mainly by the force of gravity. Thus emptying of such a diverticulum is significantly hampered, and constant retention of food content contributes not only to impaired swallowing, but also to inflammatory changes and/or ulceration in the diverticulum.

Main complaints reported by the patients include difficulties on quick swallowing of food, and sensation of retention of food in the neck during meals. When the diverticulum is small, patients try to eat slowly, drink abundantly during meals, and a gentle massage in the region of the diverticulum, which the patients perform themselves, facilitates its emptying. Endoscopic examination is very difficult and dangerous in such cases due to the possibility of puncturing of the diverticulum, to which the end of the device falls notoriously and then visualization of the cervical anastomosis, which is located on the posterior-lateral wall is very difficult. However radiological examination, which reveals perfectly the diverticular dilatation of the blind stump on the neck together with the retained contrast medium seems invaluable (Fig. 7).

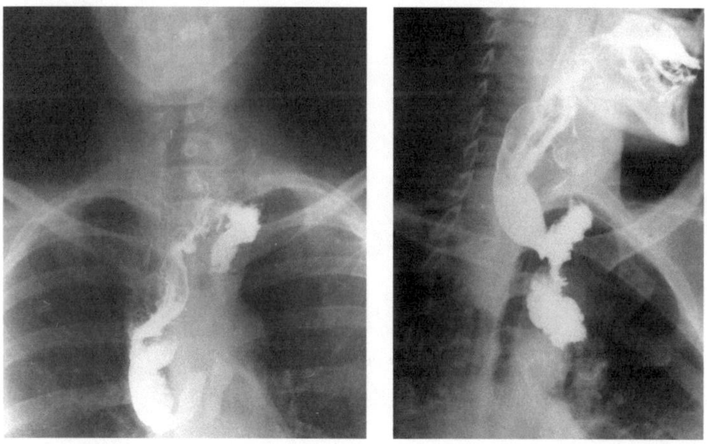

Figure 7 Radiogram of esophageal substitute from the ileum visualizing diverticulum in the region of cervical anastomosis (A-P and lateral projections)

In such cases a repair procedure in which the intestinal excess creating the diverticulum is excised is the treatment of choice. The surgical procedure is much easier in comparison to this described above for cicatrical anastomotic stenosis in the cervical region. The principle of a precise preparation of the cephalic portion of the graft has to be maintained definitely, the pedicle has to be identified, and the diverticulum excised safely without injuring the pedicle. Major difficulties may occur in cases of large diverticula, as they often are arranged in such a way that their apices descend low towards the mediastinum and their preparation may cause significant problems, the more that diverticular walls, constantly stretched by retaining saliva and food, become significantly thinner. In such cases delicacy and special care during preparation of the diverticulum and well recognition of the topographic conditions are mandatory.

2.2.3. Pleural hernia of the esophageal substitute

Pleural hernias originate as a consequence of unnoticed even small injury to the mediastinal pleura at the stage of preparation of the retrosternal canal. They occur more commonly on the right side, left-sided hernias are rare. The reason lies in the topography of the anterior mediastinum.

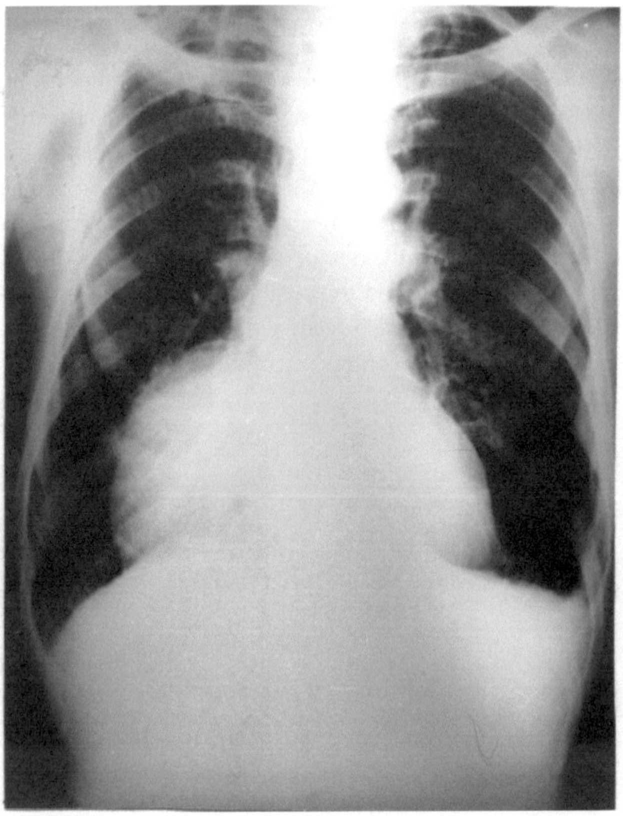

Figure 8 Radiogram of patient's chest with a visible right pleural hernia of the esophageal substitute – visible shadowing of the lower right lung (A-P projection)

The mediastinum is limited in front by the sternum and partly by the costal cartilage, in behind – by the spinal column, and on the sides – by the right and left mediastinal pleura. The anterior border of the right pleura runs behind the sternum, reaches the midline, and even passes it on the left, to pass into the lower border at the level of VI intercostals space. The anterior border of the left pleura, running downwards, reaches the cartilage of the IV rib, next it deviates to the left, crosses the V rib cartilage and reaches the VI rib, where passes to the lower border. The right and the left mediastinal pleuras approach each other at the level of the III –IV costal cartilage. Thus two free triangular interpleural spaces are created – the superior and the inferior ones. The superior space is filled with adipose tissue and the remains of the glandula thymi, while the inferior one is filled with the pericardium, which at the level of costal cartilages at the site of their sternal attachment, is not covered with the pleura. For this reason on formation of the retrosternal canal, the pleura is more often injured on the right side.

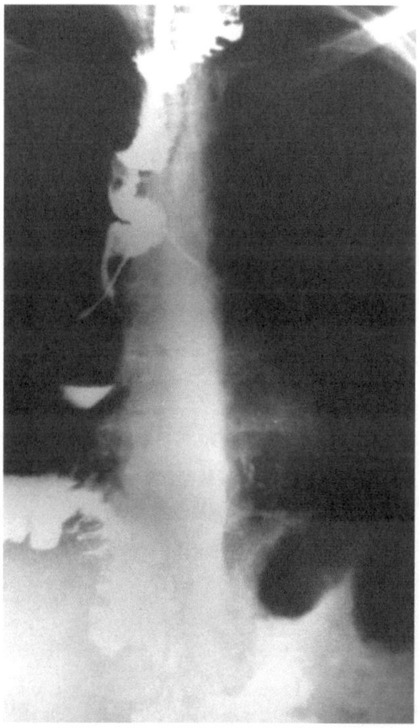

Figure 9 Radiogram of esophageal substitute from the ileum and right colon (A-P projection). Distal portion of the esophageal substitute filled with contrast medium visible in the right pleural cavity (right pleural hernia)

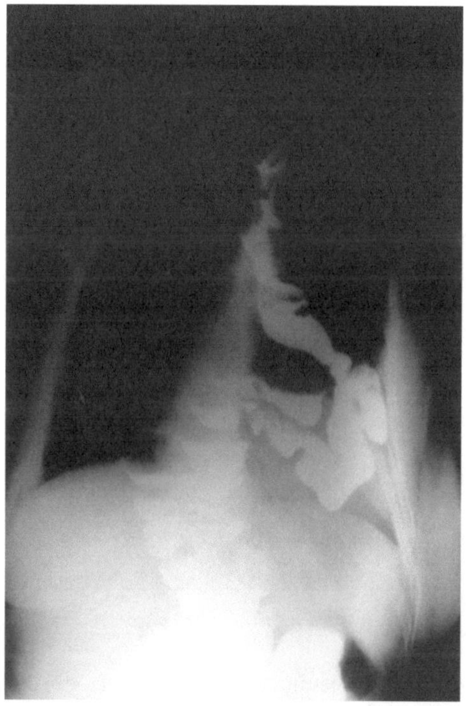

Figure 10 Radiogram of esophageal substitute from the ileum and right colon (A-P projection). Distal portion of the esophageal substitute filled with contrast medium visible in the left pleural cavity (left pleural hernia)

Initially pleural hernia is asymptomatic. However chest pain, which aggravates on meals, especially profuse, may set in with time. The pain often of a distending character is accompanied by sensation of dyspnoea and difficulties on breathing. Patients often assume lying position on the side contralateral to the hernia, what brings relief, as facilitates intestinal emptying, they also consume smaller portions of meals in fear of complaints.

Physical examination, especially auscultation often reveals distinct weakening of the alveolar murmur in the lower lungs, often associated with audible rumbling and flowing on the side of the hernia. Due to permanent limitation of the size of meals, the patients may with time develop undernourishment and anaemia, and permanently impaired lung ventilation contributes to oxygen deficiency, what may be easily confirmed on gasometry and spirometric evaluation. Chest x-ray reveals shadowing of the pulmonary field on the side of the hernia as well as shadow of the esophageal substitute filled with air with level of fluid (Fig. 8). The image is completed with contrast examination of the upper gastrointestinal series (Fig. 9, 10).

Examination with contrast medium determines not only the size of the hernia, but also evaluates passage of the contrast medium and duration of its retention in the intestinal segment in the hernia. Endoscopic examination is as much significant in these cases as it enables identification of possible inflammatory conditions and determination of their severity in the intestinal segment involved in the hernia, what may be extremely valuable and provides basis to implement supportive pharmacotherapy.

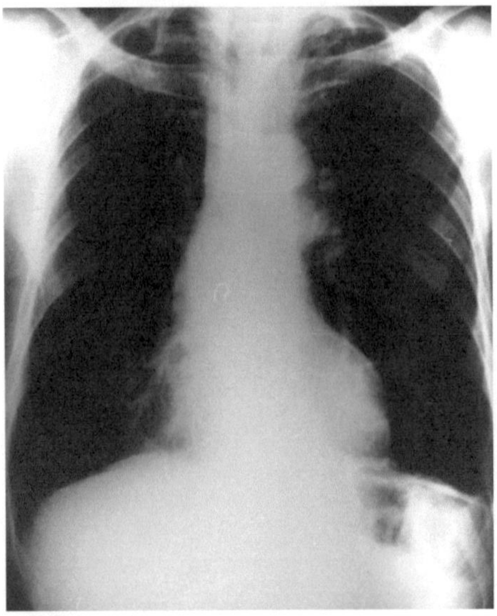

Figure 11 Chest x-ray after repair surgery of the right pleural hernia of the esophageal substitute (A-P projection)

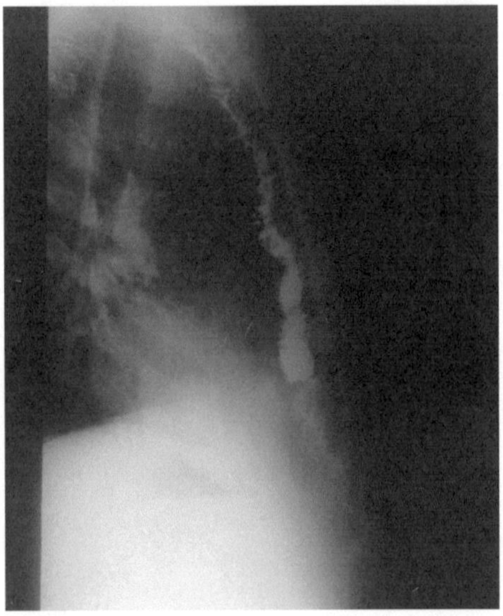

Figure 12 Radiogram of the esophageal substitute after repair surgery of the right pleural hernia (lateral projection)

The only effective therapy for pleural hernia is a repair surgery. Such operations belong to extremely difficult procedures, performed in topographic conditions which have been altered completely by the reconstructive surgery and the presence of the hernia. Moreover, a fear not to damage the graft's vascular pedicle exacerbates hazards of the operation. Generally speaking, the repair procedure consists in opening of the abdominal cavity from upper midline incision prolonged onto the sternum, preparation of the intestinal loop from the pleural cavity, its placement and stabilization in the anterior mediastinum and closure of the hernia ring. The most effective modality to achieve this is to prepare the intestinal loop, excise its excess and perform anastomosis reconstructing continuity of the graft. The most hazardous stage of the repair procedure is the preparation of the caudal segment of the esophageal substitute, which usually adheres firmly to the sternum, and especially its pedicle. A longitudinal incision of the sternum in the lower part often proves helpful, as it facilitates separation of the graft and provides access to the hernia. On completion of this stage of the procedure, the hernia has to be managed and its recurrences prevented. Removal of the intestinal loop from the pleural cavity does not usually pose any problems, as it is generally surrounded by soft, delicate adhesions, which can be easily released. However the pedicle is surrounded by solid and tough adhesions, the separation of which at any cost may bring an unfavourable outcome as far as vitality of the graft is concerned. Thus in cases of a significant excess of the intestinal loop, which forms the hernia, after getting the intestine out of the pleural cavity and bringing it to the anterior mediastinum, it is more advantageous to perform intestine-to-intestine anastomosis within the elongated loop, what shall facilitate emptying of the esophageal substitute, improve passage, and at the same time, prevent recurrences thanks to stabilization of the intestine by the performed anastomosis (Fig. 11, 12).

In extreme cases, when hernia reaches significant size, and its removal from the pleural cavity is associated with an inevitable injury to the pedicle, it is better to give up and abandon the idea of bringing the intestinal loop to the mediastinum, instead, a relatively broad additional intestinal anastomosis within the elongated loop should suffice. Such a management facilitates passage and improves emptying of the esophageal substitute and definitely ameliorates the symptoms of hernia.

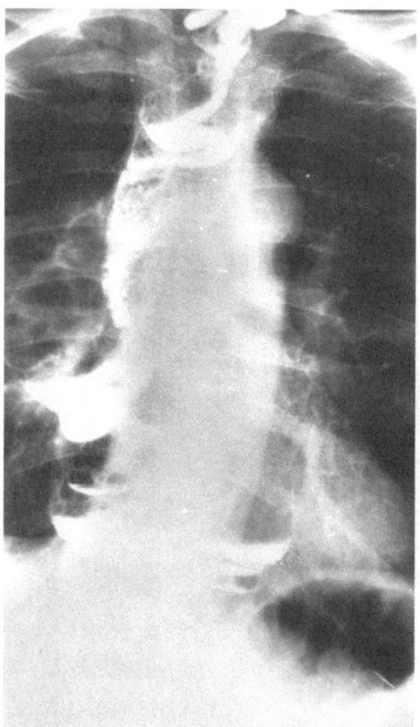

Figure 13 Radiogram of obstruction of the esophageal substitute from the colon due to right pleural hernia (A-P projection). The examination was performed with aqueous solution of contrast medium

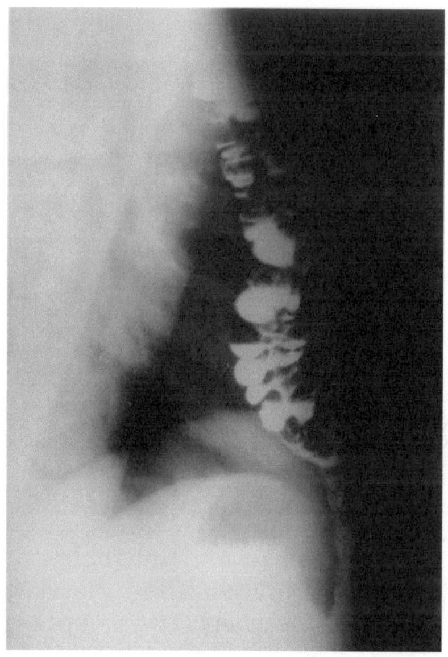

Figure 14 Radiogram of the same patient after repair surgery of the esophageal substitute occlussion (lateral projection)

Acute obstruction of the esophageal substitute is a serious, but extremely rare complication of pleural hernia. This complication may occur as a result of torsion of the elongated intestinal loop along its axis (Fig. 13). The situation requires immediate, lifesaving surgical intervention, and the procedure is extremely difficult and there are no conventions for the surgical procedure (Fig. 14). In extreme cases, when volvulus resulted in development of necrosis, the necrotic segment has to be excised and the procedure should follow steps described in the chapter:" Necrosis of a part or a whole intestinal graft".

2.2.4. Complications associated with reflux to the esophageal substitute

After reconstructive operations, when the barrier function of the cardia has been abolished, reflux of the gastric content to the esophageal substitute is very common. The mucous membrane of the intestine, which forms the esophageal substitute, is completely non-resistant to acid gastric content and undergoes inflammatory changes of various severity – from irritation and mild inflammation to haemorrhagic inflammations and ulcerations, which may in turn even lead to life threatening conditions. Clinical experience shows that the changes more often occur in esophageal substitutes from colon than those from the small intestine, which have vivid and unidirectional peristalsis, what not only accelerates the passage, but also protects against reflux. Additional barrier is provided by a long abdominal portion of the esophageal substitute anastomosed to the prepyloric part of the stomach. Another method of reflux prevention is provided by effective patency of the pylorus. It should be remembered in case of esophageal reconstructions of post-burn scars in the pyloric part of the stomach and after esophageal resections due to cancer, when the anterior and posterior trunks of the vagus nerve were cut. Restoration of gastric patency should be performed prior to esophageal reconstruction. Less patent pylorus facilitates reflux to the esophageal substitute, which, in the region of anastomosis with the stomach, is deprived of any barrier mechanism. The complaints are relieved after operation of restoration of pyloric patency (Fig. 15,16).

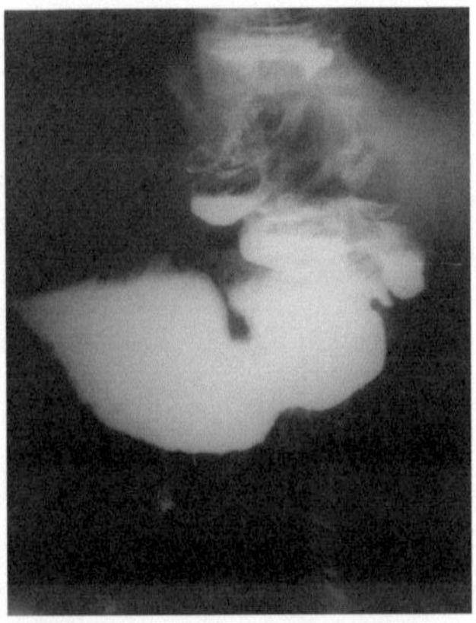

Figure 15 Radiogram of the stomach and distal portion of the esophageal substitute from the colon (A-P projection). Visible narrowing of the pylorus and deposition of contrast medium in the stomach and esophageal substitute

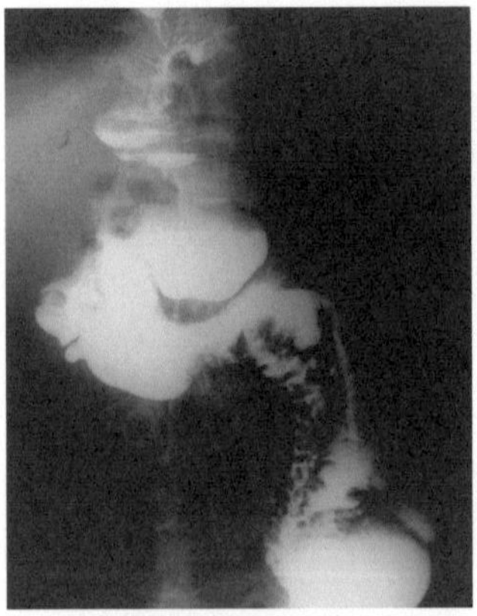

Figure 16 Radiogram of the stomach and distal portion of the esophageal substitute in the same patient after surgical restoration of gastric patency - gastro-enteroanastomosis antecolica with entero-enteroanastomosis modo Braun (A-P projection)

Prolonged reflux to the esophageal substitute leads to the development of inflammatory changes, ulcerations, haemorrhagic changes and even cicatrical stenosis.

The clinical picture of reflux is characterized by pain of retrosternal location. It may be accompanied by acid belching, sensation of squeezing, burning and tearing behind the sternum, especially after big, heavy or spicy meals. The use of neutralizing agents and eating more often light meals in smaller portions brings relief.

In order to make the diagnosis, apart from radiological evaluation, endoscopic examinations with a biopsy are very useful as they enable determination of the severity of inflammatory changes in the esophageal substitute and rule out possible neoplastic changes (Fig. 17, 18, 19, 20).

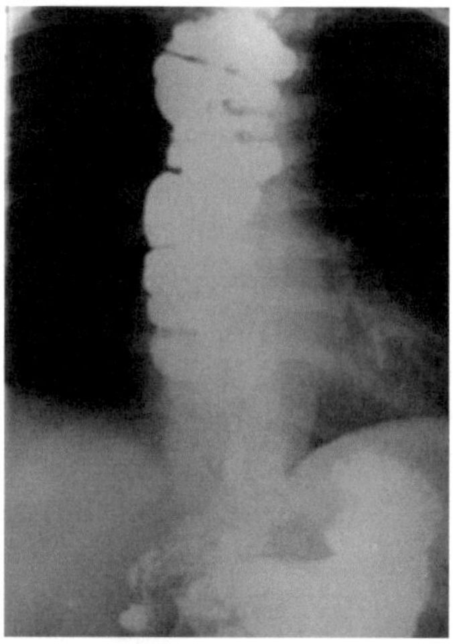

Figure 17 Radiological image of a massive reflux to the esophageal substitute from the colon in Trenelenburg's position (A-P projection)

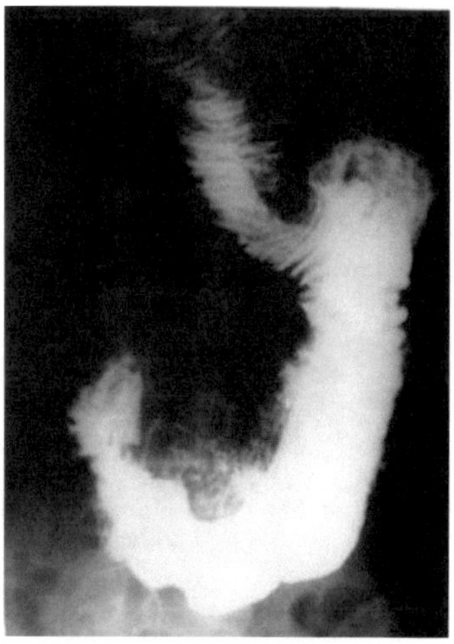

Figure 18 Radiological image of a massive reflux to the esophageal substitute from the colon visible in Trendelenburg's position, resulting from anastomosis of a distal portion of the graft with the fundus of the stomach (A-P projection)

The use of endoscopy permits to differentiate individual stages of the disease and institute adequate conservative therapy as well as evaluates the efficacy of the applied therapy.

Conservative treatment is effective with prokinetic drugs and agents protecting the mucous membrane in combination with proton pump inhibitors (PPI). In few cases healing of the inflammatory changes or ulcerations may lead to cicatrical stenosis of the distal portion of the esophageal substitute, which require complicated repair procedures together with partial excision of the distal portion of the graft and a consecutive necessity to reconstruct the continuity of the esophageal substitute by means of a pedicled insertion from the jejunum or omega-shaped jejunal loop (Fig. 21, 22, 23, 24, 25).

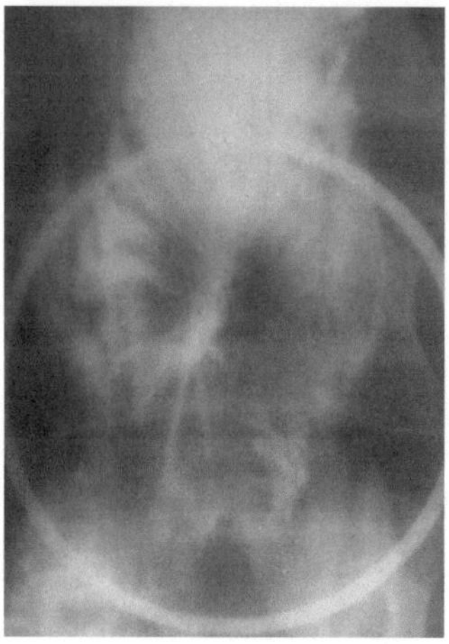

Figure 19 Radiogram imaging ulcer in a distal portion of the esophageal substitute from the colon (A-P projection)

2.2.5. Benign and malignant tumours of the esophageal substitute

Both, benign and malignant tumours of the esophageal substitute are rare and in there are only single case reports in literature. Reasons facilitating such changes in the esophageal substitute undoubtedly include an altered function of the small or large intestine which it starts to perform as an esophageal substitute. In the esophageal substitute the intestinal mucous membrane, permanently exposed to direct effect of food and contained in it chemicals, high temperature of ingested meals, and quite often – reflux, easily undergoes changes, which may become a background for neoplastic processes.

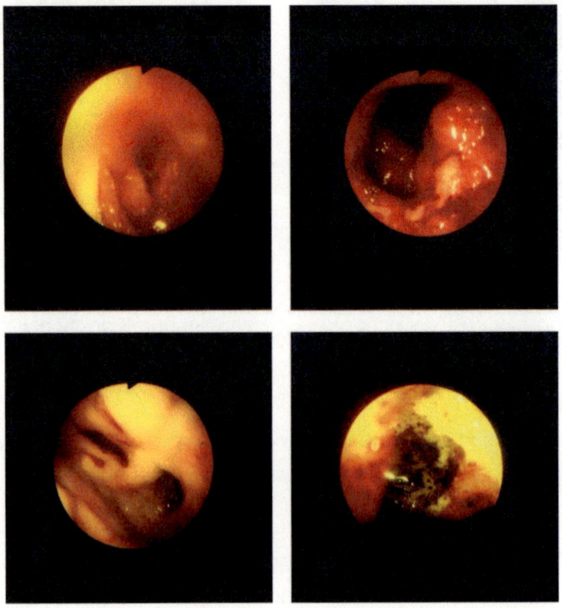

Figure 20 Endoscopic pictures imaging various stages of reflux-induced inflammation of the esophageal substitute from the colon – from inflammatory changes to haemorrhagic ulcerations

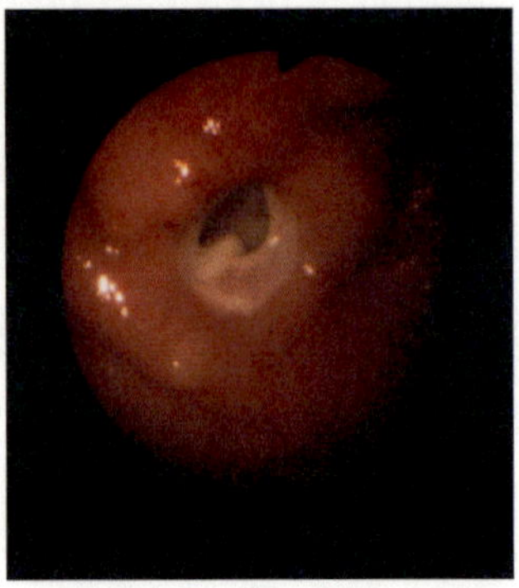

Figure 21 Endoscopic image of reflux-induced cicatrical lesions in the esophageal substitute from the colon

Polyps constitute one of better recognized precancerous conditions of the gastrointestinal tract. Polyps require resection and histopathological evaluation is indispensable, which decides whether there was a neoplastic transformation within the polyp. The fact that many disorders and conditions within the colon are asymptomatic for a long time is unquestionable. For this reason prior to reconstructive procedure endoscopic evaluation of the colon is mandatory. Moreover, periodic endoscopic examinations of patients after esophageal reconstructions with the colon should be a rule (Fig. 24). It enables detection and excision of possible polyps in the esophageal substitute, what prevents their malignant transformation, which, if occur, may require removal of the whole esophageal substitute (Fig. 26, 27).

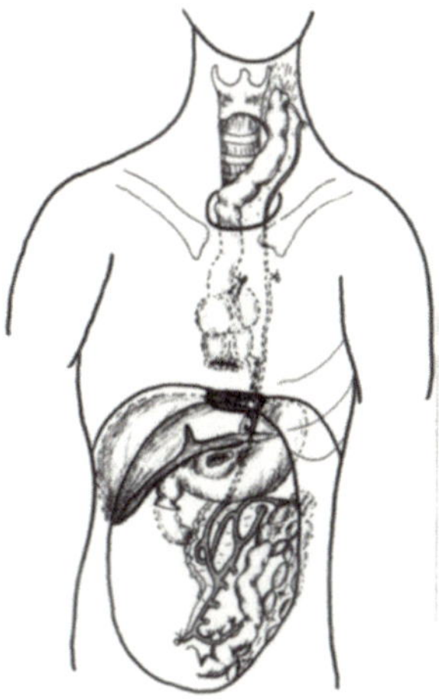

Figure 22 Diagram illustrating resection of distal portion of the esophageal substitute from the colon. Visible maintained continuity of the vascular pedicle

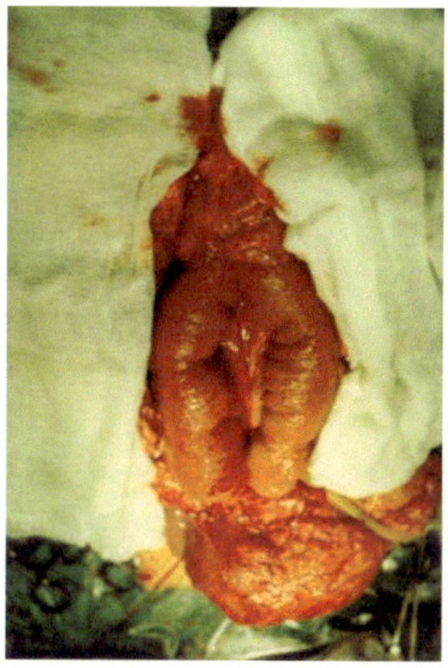

Figure 23 Intraoperative image of an omega-type insertion from the jejunum after resection of a distal portion of the esophageal substitute from the colon due to reflux-associated cicatrical stenosis

During endoscopic removal of polyps in the esophageal substitute, it should be remembered that injury to the wall may result in puncturing the intestine and life threatening complications. For these reasons the procedure should be performed in the endoscopy centre familiar with the problems of endoscopy of esophageal substitutes.

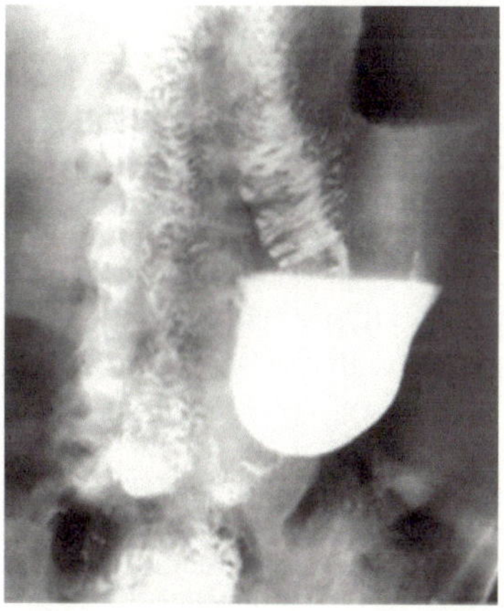

Figure 24 Radiogram of an omega-type insertion from the jejunum after resection of a distal portion of the esophageal substitute from the colon due to reflux-associated cicatrical stenosis

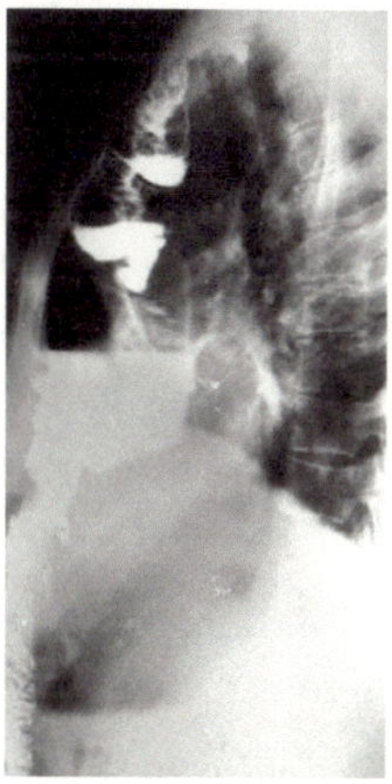

Figure 25 Radiogram of a pedicled insertion from the jejunum after resection of a distal portion of the esophageal substitute from the colon due to reflux-associated cicatrical stenosis

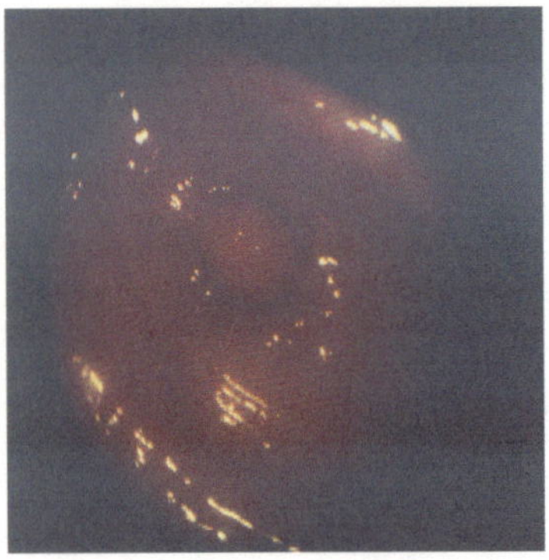

Figure 26 Endoscopic image of polyp in the esophageal substitute from the colon

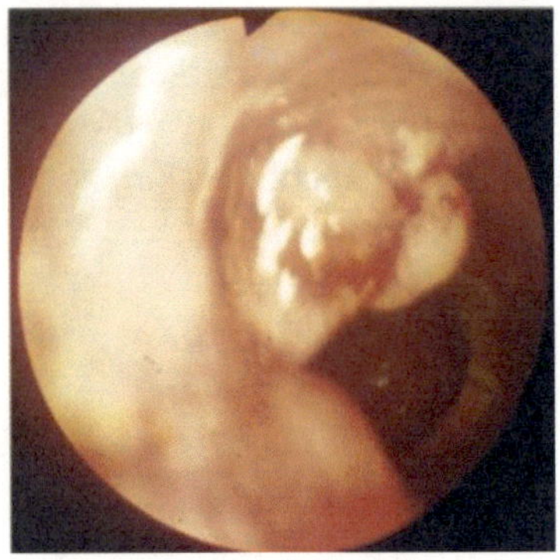

Figure 27 Endoscopic image of cancer in the esophageal substitute 30 years after esophageal reconstruction

Recapitulating the above presented early complications after esophageal reconstruction and disorders of the esophageal substitutes, it should be emphasized that patients after such procedures should be permanently followed up in specialized centres. Only then can they use indispensable information, and in case of any complaints, may count on periodic check up examinations, and if required – expert assistance and medical care.

3. References

[1] Buntain WL, Payne WS, Lynn HB. Esophageal reconstruction for benign disease: long term appraisal. Am Surg 1980, 46: 67-79.

[2] Aghaji MA, Chukwu CO. Oesophageal replacement in adult Nigerians with corrosive oesophageal strictures. Intern Surg 1993, 78: 189-192.

[3] Cerfolio RJ, Allen MS, Deschamps C, Trastek VF, Pairolero PC. Esophageal replacement by colon interposition. Ann Thorac Surg 1995, 59: 1382-1384.

[4] Cusick EL, Batchelor AAG, Spicer RD. Development of a technique for jejunal interposition in long-gap esophageal atresia. J Pediatr Surg 1993, 28: 990-994.

[5] Hirabayashi S, Miyata M, Shoji M, Shibusawa H. Reconstruction of the thoracic esophagus, with extended jejunum used as a substitute, with the aid of microvascular anastomosis. Surgery 1993, 113: 515-519.

[6] Kato H, Kuriki A, Kamei Y, Kamei Y, Torini S. Free inrathoracic jejunal transfer for thoracic oesophageal reconstruction: a case report. Br J Plast Surg 1995, 48: 11-13.

[7] Della Casa U, Picchio M, Passaro U, Lombardi A, Ramacciato G, Amodio PM, Paolini A. Esophago-jejuno-gastroplasty in treatment of peptic stenosis of the esophagus. Minerva Chir 1997, 52: 705-712.

[8] Chen HC, Tang YB. Microsurgical reconstruction of the esophagus. Semin Surg Oncol 2000, 19: 235-245.

[9] Wallentin RS, Sorensen HB, Bundgaard T, Pahle E, Nordsmark M, Pilegaard H. Reconstruction using free jejunal transfer after resection of cancer of the upper oesophagus. Dan Med Bull 2010, 57: A4164.

[10] Yasuda T, Shiozaki H. Esophageal reconstruction using a pedicled jejunum with microvascular augmentation. Ann Thorac Cardiovasc Surg 2011, 17: 103-109.

[11] Poh M, Selber JC, Skoracki R, Walsh GL, Yu P. Technical challenges of total esophageal reconstruction using a supercharge jejunal flap. Ann Surg 2011, 253: 1122-1129.

[12] Bothereau H, Munoz-Bongrand N, Lambert B, Montemagno S, Cattan P, Sarfati E. Esophageal reconstruction after caustic injury: is there still a place for right coloplasty? Am J Surg 2007, 193: 660-664.

[13] Knezević JD, Radovanović NS, Simić AP, Kotarac MM, Skrobić OM, Konstantinović ND, Pesko PH. Colon interposition in the treatment of esophageal caustic strictures: 40 years of experience. Dis Esophagus 2007, 20: 530-534.

[14] Yasuda T, Shiozaki H. Esophageal reconstruction with colon tissue. Surg Today 2011, 41: 745-753.

[15] Chernousov AF, Adrianov VA, Bogopolskii PM, Voronov ME. Choice of esophageal plastic surgery. Vestn Ross Akad Med Nauk 1997, 9: 21-25.

[16] Picchio M, Lombardi A, Zolovkins A, Della Casa U, Paolini A, Fegiz G, Mihelson M. Jejunal interposition for peptic stenosis of the esophagus following esophagomyotomy for achalasia. Int Surg 1997, 82: 198-200.

[17] Jacob L, Rabary O, Boudaoud S, Payen D, Sarfati E, Gossot D, Rolland E, Eurin B, Celerier M. Usefulness of perioperative pulsed Doppler flowmetry in predicting postoperative local ischaemic complications after ileocolic esophagoplasty. J Thorac Cardiovasc Surg 1992, 104: 385-389.

[18] Vereczkei A, Rozsos I, Horvath OP. Subacute ischemic lesions in jejunal loops used for esophageal reconstruction. Dis Esophagus 1998, 11: 194-197.

[19] Nicks R. Colonic replacement of the oesophagus. Some observations on infarction and wound leakage. Br J Surg 1967, 54: 124-128.

[20] Strutyńska-Karpińska M. Causes of blood perfusion disturbances in pedunculated intestinal grafts employed in reconstructive procedures of the esophagus. Pol Przeg Chir 1993, 65: 1185-1190.

[21] Strutyńska-Karpińska M. Retrosternal canal in reconstructive procedures of the entire esophagus. Pol Przegl Chir 1997;69: 1191-1196.

[22] Xia J, Peng Y, Huang J. Cheng BC, Wang ZW. Prevention and treatment of anastomotic leakage and intestinal ischemia after esophageal replacement with colon. Chinese J Gastrointest Surg 2009, 12: 17-19.

[23] Strutyńska-Karpińska M. Early postoperative complications in reconstructive operations of the esophagus. Pol Przeg Chir 1997, 69: 677-685.

[24] Nienartowicz M, Strutyńska-Karpińska M, Śliwa B. A novel method of reconstructive surgery of the esophagus. Adv Clin Exp Med, 2008, 17: 583-585.

[25] Lorentz T, Fok M, Wong J. Anastomotic leakage after resection and bypass for esophageal cancer: lessons learned from the past. World J Surg 1989, 13: 472-477.

[26] Strutyńska-Karpińska M. Frequency of cervical anastomotic leaks after various types of oesophagoplasty – a retrospective study. Adv Clin Exp Med 2002, 11: 473-479.

[27] Nienartowicz M., Nienartowicz E., Grabowski K., Strutyńska-Karpińska M., Błaszczuk J., Szelachowski P. Preoperative evaluation of the upper section of the retrosternal tunnel in esophageal reconstruction procedures. Adv Clin Exp Med 2009, 18: 159-162.

[28] Vereczkei A, Varga G, Poto L, Horvath OP. Management of corrosive injuries of the esophagus. Acta Chir Hung 1999, 38: 119-122.

[29] de Jong AL, Macdonald R, Ein S, Forte V, Turner A. Corrosive esophagitis in children: a 30-year review. Int J Pediatr Otolaryngol 2001, 57: 203-211.

[30] Wu MH, Tseng YT, Lin MY, Lai WW. Esophageal reconstruction for hypopharyngoesophageal strictures after corrosive injury. Eur J Cardiothorac Surg 2001, 19: 400-405.

[31] Mutaf O, Ozok G, Avanoglu A. Oesophagoplasty in the treatment of caustic oesophageal strictures in children. Br J Surg 1995, 82: 644-646.

[32] Neville WE, Najem AZ. Colon replacement of the esophagus for congenital and benign disease. Ann Thorac Surg 1983, 36: 626-633.

[33] Postlethwait RW. Colonic interposiotion for esophageal substitution. Surg Gynecol Obst 1983, 156: 377-383.

[34] Ribet M, Barrat C. Colonic esophagoplasty for benign lesions. Ann Chir 1995, 49: 133-137.

[35] Scharli AF. Esophageal reconstruction by elongation of the lesser gastric curvature. Surg Childh Intern 1999, 7: 170-173.

[36] Stefan H. Esophageal replacement using large intestine in children. Rozhl V Chir 1992, 71: 530-535.

[37] Higton DIR, Ford IJ. Dysphagia following colon pedicle grafts. Br J Surg 1970, 57: 825-828.

[38] Cheng BC, Xia J, Liu XP, Mao ZF, Zeng ZY, Huang J, Xiao YG, Wang TS, Hu H, Wu XJ. Observation on the long-term complications after esophageal replacement with colon. Zhonghua Wai Ke Za Zhi 2007, 45: 118-120.

[39] De Delva PE, Morse CR, Austen WG Jr, Gaissert HA, Lanuti M, Wain JC, Wright CD, Mathisen DJ. Surgical management of failed colon interposition. Eur J Cardiothorac Surg. 2008, 34: 432-437.

[40] Cigna E, Ozkan O, Chen HC. Dysphagia [corrected] due to solitary jejunal diverticulum after free jejunal transfer for reconstruction of the cervical oesophagus. J Plast Reconstr Aesthet Surg 2006, 59: 874-877.

[41] Strutyńska-Karpińska M, Ciesielska A, Błaszczuk J, Wierzbicki J, Zielony A, Taboła R. Evaluation of types of cervical anastomoses in oesophageal reconstructive surgery. Adv Clin Exp Med 2002, 11: 445-450.

[42] Tuszewski F. The radiologic appearance of the reconstructed esophagus. Acta Radiol Scand 1972, 12: 193-197.

[43] Isolauri J, Reinikainen P, Markkula H. Functional evaluation of intersopsed colon in esophagus. Manometric and 24-hour ph observations. Acta Chir Scand 1987, 153: 21-24.

[44] Isolauri J, Paakkala T, Arajarvi P, Markkula H. Colon interposition. Long-term radiographic results. Eur J Radiol 1987, 7: 248-252.

[45] Eleftheriadis E, Dadoukis J, Kotzampassi K, Aletras H. Long-term results after esophagoplasty with colon: An endoskopic study. Int Surg 1987, 72: 11-12.

[46] Isolauri J, Helin H, Markkula H. Colon interposition for esophageal disease: histologic findings of colonic mucosa after a follow-up of five months to 15 years. Am J Gastroenterol 1991, 86: 277-280.

[47] Young MM, Deschamps C, Trastek VF, Allen MS, Miller DL, Schleck CD, Pairolero PC. Esophageal reconstruction for benign disease: early morbidity, mortality, and functional results. Ann Thorac Surg 2000, 70: 1651-1655.

[48] Dantas RO, Mamede RCH. Motility of the transverse colon used for esophageal replacement. J Clin Gastroenterol 2002, 34: 225-228.

[49] Milnerowicz S, Strutyńska-Karpińska M, Grabowski K, Lewandowski A. Long term results after esophagoplasty with the large and small bowel. Surg Childh Intern 1999, 7: 197-199.

[50] Grabowski K, Bernat M, Strutyńska M, Lewandowski A. Problems in diagnosing and treatment of complication of peptic ulcer in artificial oesophagus. Pol Przeg Chir 1990, 62: 523-526.

[51] Gossot D, Lefebvre JF. Ischaemic atrophy of the cervical portion of a substernal colonic transplant: successful reconstruction using a synthetic resorbable tube. Br J Surg 1988, 75: 801-802.

[52] Grabowski K, Lewandowski A, Moroń K, Strutyńska-Karpińska M, Błaszczuk J, Machała R. Pleural hernia of an esophageal graft-late postoperative complication. Wiad Lek. 1997, 50 Suppl 1, 1:339-343.

[53] Kok VK. Perforation of a substernal interposed ileocolon caused by right thoracic herniation. Asian Cardoivasc Thorac Ann 2007, 15: 515-517.

[54] Strutyńska-Karpińska M, Lewandowski A, Knast W, Markocka-Maczka K, Czapla L, Błaszczuk J. Comparative evaluation of postoperative complication in the reconstructive surgery of the esophagus. Wiad Lek. 1999, 52:367-372.

[55] Grabowski K, Błaszczuk J, Strutyńska-Karpińska M. Complications and treatment of esophagi constructed from bowel grafts. Pol Przgl Chir 2002, 74: 23-30.

[56] Fancioni F, De Giacomo T, Jo Filice M, Anile M, Diso D, Venuta F, Coloni GF. Surgical treatment of redundancy after retrosternal esophagocoloplasty. Minerva Chir 2009, 64: 317-319.

[57] Milnerowicz S, Grabowski K, Strutyńska-Karpińska M, Knast W. Gastroesophageal reflux after reconstruction of the esophagus with colon interposition. Wiad Lek. 1997, 50 Suppl 1, 1:322-325.

[58] Maurer SV, Estremadoyro V, Reinberg O. Evaluation of an antireflux procedure for colonic interposition in pediatric esophageal replacements. J Pediatr Surg 2011, 46: 594-600.

[59] Yano M, Motoori M, Tanaka K, Kishi K, Miyashiro I, Shingai T, Gotoh K, Noura S, Takahashi H, Yamada T, Ohue M, Ohigashi H, Ishikawa O. Prevention of gastroduodenal content reflux and delayed gastric emptying after esophagectomy: gastric tube reconstruction with duodenal diversion plus Roux-en-Y anastomosis. Dis Esophagus 2011 doi: 10.1111/j. 1442-2050.2011.011229.

[60] Ngan SYK, Wong J: Lenghts of different routes for esophageal replacement. J Thorac Cardiovasc Surg 1986, 91: 790-792.

[61] Rakić S, Diuranović S: Lenghts of different routes for esophageal replacement in a white population. J Thorac Cardiovasc Surg 1993;105: 1122.

[62] Chien KY, Wang PY, Lu KS. Esophagoplasty for corrosive stricture of the esophagus: an analysis of 60 cases. Ann Surg 1974, 197: 510-515.

[63] Zadorozhnyi AA, Baidala PG. Reconstructive operations on the artificial esophagus. Vestn Khir Im II Grek 1993, 151: 78-81.

[64] Keminger K, Roka R. Complications after esophageal replacement. Zentralbl Chir 1997, 102: 1136-1147.

[65] Schumpelick V, Dreuw B, Ophoff K, Fass J. Esophageal - replacement indications, technique, results. Leber Magen Darm 1995, 25: 21-26.

[66] Moreno-Osset E, Tomas-Ridocci M, Paris F, Mora F, Garcia-Zarza A, Molina R, Pastor J, Benager A. Motor activity of esophageal substitute (stomach, jejunal, and colon segments). Ann Thorac Surg 1986, 41: 515-519.

[67] Jezioro Z. Etiopathogenesis of the regurgitation of gastric contents after esophagoplasty with the use of the large intestine. Pol Przegl Chir 1967, 39: 912-919.

[68] Jezioro Z, Bernat M, Piegza S, Zimmer Z. Hemorrhagic, peptic esophagitis of an esophagus made from the colon. Pol Przegl Chir. 1967, 39: 1-6.

[69] Miller H, Lam KH, Ong GB. Observations of pressure waves in stomach, jejunal, and colonic loops used to replace the esophagus. Surg 1975, 78: 543-551.

[70] Rode H, Cywes S, Millar AJ, Davies MR. Colonic replacement in children – functional results. Z Kinderchir 1986, 41: 201-205.

[71] Grabowski K, Błaszczuk J, Woźniak S, Temler M, Szelachowski P. The second reconstructive operation of the esophagus. Wiad Lek 2000, 53: 98-103.

[72] Chernousov AF, Ruchkin DV, Chernousov FA, Kebedov MM. Experience in repeated esophagoplasty. Khirurgia (Mosk) 2005, 5: 14-19.

[73] Okazaki M, Asato H, Takushima A, Nakatsuka T, Ueda K, Harii K. Secondary reconstruction of failed esophageal reconstruction. Ann Plast Surg 2005, 54: 530-537.

[74] Parmar JM, Prober C, Clarke DB, Temple JG. Colopericardial and colo-caval fistula. Late complication of colon interposition. Eur J Cardiothorac Surg 1989, 3: 371-372.

[75] Kotsis L, Krisár Z, Orbán K, Csekeö A. Late complications of coloesophagoplasty and long-term features of adaptation. Surgery 2002, 21: 79-83.

[76] Cherki S, Mabrut JY, Adham M, De La Roche E, Ducerf C, Gouillat C, Berard P, Baulieux J. Reinterventions for complication and defect of coloesophagoplasty. Ann Chir 2005, 130: 242-248.

[77] Oki M, Asato H, Suzuki Y, Umekawa K, Takushima A, Okazaki M, Harii K. Salvage reconstruction of the oesophagus: a retrospective study of 15 cases. J Plast Reconstr Aesthet Surg 2010, 63: 589-597.

[78] McLarty AJ, Deschamps C, TrastekVF, Allen MS, Pairolero PC, Harmsen WS. Esophageal resection for cancer of the esophagus: long-term function and quality of life. Ann Thorac Surg 1997, 63: 1568-1572.

[79] Cseke L, Horvath OP. Indications, new surgical technique and results of colon interposition or bypass in esophageal surgery. Acta Chir Hung 1997, 36: 49-50.

[80] Rosinska T, Bernat M, Bader O, Markowska A, Strutynska M. Dumping syndrome and reactive hypoglycemia in a patient following esophagoplasty and methods of treatment. Zentralbl Chir. 1987, 112: 320-326.

[81] Jezioro Z. Functional results and delayed complications following retrosternal surgery producing and esophagus from large intestine by my own method, 1950-1970. Pol Przeg Chir 1977, 49: 1199-1205.

[82] Skinner DB. Esophageal reconstruction. Am J Surg 1980, 139: 810-814.

[83] Bernat M. Usefulness of the jejunum in fashioning whole retrosternal esophagus anastomosed with larynx. Pol Przeg Chir 1977, 49: 1147-1153.

[84] Calleja IJ, Moreno E, Santoyo J, Gomez M, Navalon J, Atrias J, Castellanos G, Solis JA. Long esophagoplasty: functional study. Hepatogastroenterology 1988, 35: 279-284.

[85] Thomas P, Giudicelli R, Fuentes P, Reboud E. Technique and results of colonic esophagoplasties. Ann Chir 1996, 50: 106-120.

[86] Svanes K, Stangeland L, Viste A, Varhang JE, Groubech JE, Soreide O. Morbidity, ability to swallow, and survival, after oesophagectomy for cancer. Europ J Surg 1995, 161: 669-675.

[87] Nardi GL, Glotzer DS. Anastomosis ulcer of the colon following colonic replacement of the esophagus. Ann Surg 1960, 152: 10-12.

[88] Isolauri J, Markkula H. Reccurent ulceration and colopericardiac fistula as late complications of colon interposition. Ann Thorac Surg 1987, 44: 84-85.

[89] Jezioro Z, Zimmer Z, Piegza S. Cancer of the artificial esophagus: partial resection and esophageal replacement by transplant from the ileum. Surgery 1960, 48: 828-837.

[90] Goldsmith HS, Beattie EJ. Malignant villous tumor in a colon bypass. Ann Thorac Surg 1968, 167: 98-100.

[91] Haerr RW, Higgins EM, Seymore CH, el-Mahdi AM. Adenocarcinoma arising in a colonic interposition following resection of squamous cell oesophageal cancer. Cancer 1987, 60: 2304-2307.

[92] Houghton AD, Jourdan M, Mc Coll I. Dukes A carcinoma after colonic interposition for oesophageal stricture. Gut 1989, 30: 880-881.

[93] Goyal M, Bang DH, Cohen LE. Adenocarcinoma arising in interposed colon: report of a case. Dis Colon Rectum 2000, 43: 555-558.

[94] Novotny AR, Florack G, Becker K, Siewert JR. Esophageal replacement by Lexer' s esophagoplasty: adenocarcinoma as late complication. Ann Thorac Surg 2005, 80: 1122-1124.

[95] Hwang HJ, Song KH, Youn YH, Kwon JE, Kim H, Chung JB, Lee YC. A case of more abundant and dysplastic adenomas in interposed colon than in native colon. Yonsei Med J 2007, 48: 1075-1078.